Quick & Easy
MEDICAL
Terminology

Quick & Easy

MEDICAL
Terminology

Peggy C. Leonard, B.A., M.T., M.Ed.

1990

W.B. SAUNDERS COMPANY

Harcourt Brace Jovanovich, Inc.

Philadelphia ■ London ■ Toronto ■ Montreal ■ Sydney ■ Tokyo

W. B. SAUNDERS COMPANY
Harcourt Brace Jovanovich, Inc.

The Curtis Center
Independence Square West
Philadelphia, PA 19106-3399

Library of Congress Cataloging-in-Publication Data

Leonard, Peggy C.
  Quick and easy medical terminology/Peggy C. Leonard.
     p.   cm.
  Includes bibliographical references.
  ISBN 0-7216-5726-5
  1. Medicine—Terminology.   I. Title.
  [DNLM: 1. Nomenclature.   W 15 L581q]
R123.L47   1990
610′.14—dc20
DNLM/DLC
for Library of Congress   89-24302
                                                                  CIP

Editor: Margaret M. Biblis
Developmental Editor: Leslie E. Hoeltzel
Designer: Bill Donnelly
Production Manager: Peter Faber
Manuscript Editor: Louise Robinson
Cover Designer: Jim Gerhart

QUICK AND EASY MEDICAL TERMINOLOGY   ISBN 0-7216-5726-5

Printed in the United States of America.

Last digit is the print number: 9   8   7   6   5   4   3   2

Preface

Quick and Easy Medical Terminology is a student-oriented book that can easily be used as self-paced material or in a structured classroom setting to provide a fast, working knowledge of medical terms. It will be useful to anyone pursuing a career in the allied health fields. It can also be helpful to persons already working in these areas who have never taken a course in medical terminology and who wish to increase their understanding and use of medical terms.

This textbook is written for those who must acquire an understanding of medical terminology in a short period, but it still enables the student to recognize and write thousands of medical terms! *Quick and Easy Medical Terminology* can be used in a short medical terminology course, or it can be studied in conjunction with courses in anatomy, physiology, or introductory medical science, and with foundation programs for careers in health or medicine, particularly those based on body systems. *Quick and Easy Medical Terminology* is based on body systems, and chapters can be studied in any order after the material in the first three orientation chapters has been learned.

The student will welcome the elimination of memorizing definitions. Instead, several word parts are given, as well as rules for using them to write medical terms and for recognizing the word parts in unfamiliar terms. Various teaching methods are used, including word association, programming, review exercises (after small, easily learned sections), and comprehensive end-of-chapter reviews that serve as self-tests. Each chapter contains substantial textual material in addition to programmed study sections, and word part lists. Pronunciation is also shown.

Helpful material is found in the appendices, such as medical abbreviations and symbols, pharmacologic terms, physician specialties, and rules for forming plurals.

I wish to thank the reviewers who offered encouragement and helpful suggestions. I also thank those at the W. B. Saunders Company whose expertise has produced a book that I am confident will be useful to those who need a quickly learned, basic vocabulary in medical terminology.

PEGGY C. LEONARD

Contents

SECTION I
Orientation 1

CHAPTER 1
Rationale Behind Quick and Easy Medical Terminology: Essential Information for Learning by This Quick and Easy
Method 3

CHAPTER 2
Using Suffixes and Combining Forms to Write Medical
Terms 11

CHAPTER 3
Using Prefixes, Suffixes, and Combining Forms to Write
Medical Terms 39

SECTION II
Body Structure and Body Systems 71

CHAPTER 4
Body Structure 73

CHAPTER 5
The Skeletal and Muscular Systems 99

CHAPTER 6
The Circulatory System 125

CHAPTER 7
The Respiratory System 149

CHAPTER 8
The Digestive System 169

CHAPTER 9
The Urinary System 189

CHAPTER 10
The Reproductive System 205

SECTION III
Review **231**

CHAPTER 11
Review of Chapters 1 to 10 233

APPENDIX I
Physician Specialties 255

APPENDIX II
Forming Plurals of Medical Words 257

APPENDIX III
Medical Abbreviations and Symbols 259

APPENDIX IV
Pharmacologic Terms, Drugs, and Use 263

APPENDIX V
Glossary of Word Parts 273

APPENDIX VI
Answers to Exercises 281

Bibliography 299

Index 301

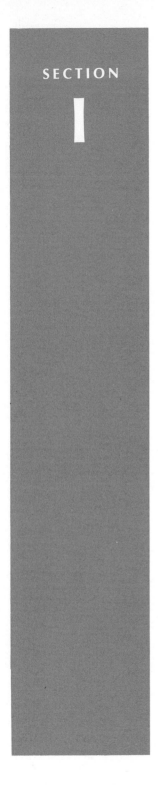

Orientation

1

Rationale Behind Quick and Easy Medical Terminology: Essential Information for Learning by This Quick and Easy Method

OBJECTIVES

After completing Chapter 1 you will be able to

1. Recognize prefixes, suffixes, and word roots as word parts used to write medical terms.
2. Demonstrate understanding of the rules for using word parts by combining them correctly to form medical terms.

OUTLINE

SIMPLIFYING DIFFICULT MEDICAL TERMS
WORD PARTS
COMBINING WORD PARTS TO WRITE MEDICAL TERMS
PRONUNCIATION OF MEDICAL TERMS
    Guide to pronunciation used in this book
    Basic rules for pronunciation

SIMPLIFYING DIFFICULT MEDICAL TERMS

The great size of a medical dictionary is evidence of the vast number of words in the medical language. **Latin** and **Greek** are the major sources of medical terms, so this offers some insight into why some people say "Medical words look like Greek to me!" The Greeks borrowed the art of writing from the Phoenicians about 850 BC. During the first century BC many Greek words were borrowed by the Romans, who adapted their spelling to Latin. Although familiarity with Greek or Latin would simplify the task of learning medical terminology, experience has shown that learning these two languages is not necessary. **What is necessary is learning relatively few word parts and recognizing them when you see them in a word.** This prevents having to memorize every new word you encounter.

The material in Chapters 1 to 3 is essential for learning medical terms, because it explains **word building** and teaches you how to divide words into their **component parts.** Subsequent chapters do not have to be studied in the sequence in which they appear in this book, but they are presented with the assumption that you have learned the material in the first three chapters. There are many **word parts** that are used to form medical terms that pertain to every body system. For example, "-itis" is a suffix that means inflammation; therefore, one will see this word part used in describing various inflammatory conditions that occur throughout the body. **No matter how eager you are to learn medical terminology pertaining to a particular body system, don't skip any of the material in the first three chapters of this book!** It is the foundation on which you will build to speak, read, and write medical terms correctly.

Correct spelling is essential because a misspelled word may give an entirely different meaning! In many cases correct spelling can also help with pronunciation. The correct pronunciation will be shown in a footnote at the bottom of the page on which the word is shown for the first time in a chapter. Learning to pronounce terms can also improve your spelling.

Writing words helps one to learn faster than simply reading them, and you will often be asked to write answers. Write an answer whenever you see a blank or a question. You are also frequently instructed to check your answer to see if it is correct. Even when you think you're sure that you know the answer, **check your answer** anyway. Sometimes we misinterpret what we read and this is an excellent way to check your understanding. Written exercises throughout each chapter get you actively involved. Comprehensive reviews at the end of each chapter can be used as self-tests to ensure that you have learned the material.

Greater retention of material occurs when students make use of various learning methods. **This book is designed for you to write in as well as to read.** In addition, some students find that pronouncing new terms aloud helps them to remember them better. A pronunciation guide is presented later in this chapter. It is not intended to be memorized but to provide general rules used in the pronunciation of medical terms and to explain the method of pronunciation used in this book.

WORD PARTS

All words have a **word root,** even ordinary words. **The word root is the main body of a word.** Compound words are sometimes composed of two word roots, as in *checkbook* (check and book). A vowel, called a **combining vowel,** is often inserted between word roots to make the word easier to pronounce, as in speed/o/meter. Speed/o is a combining form that is simply the word root *speed* plus the vowel o. **A combining form can be recognized by the diagonal slash mark before a vowel.** (The most frequently used vowel is *o*.) Cardi/o, gastr/o, and oste/o are all combining forms, but so is chol/e. In this book you will learn the combining forms for word roots.

A word root is usually accompanied by a prefix or a suffix, or sometimes by both. **A prefix is placed before a word to modify its meaning.** When written alone a prefix is usually followed by a hyphen, indicating that another word part follows the prefix. (For example, the prefix *a*-, meaning without, joined with *febrile*, which refers to fever, yields the term *afebrile*. The new term *afebrile* means without fever.)

A suffix is attached to the end of a word or word root to modify its meaning. Suffixes are joined to combining forms to write nouns, adjectives, or verbs. A suffix is usually preceded by a hyphen when the suffix is written alone, indicating that another word part needs to precede it before a complete word can be formed. (For example, -cyte is a suffix that means *cell*. Erythr/o is a combining form that means *red*. Erythr/o is joined with the suffix -cyte to obtain the new term *erythrocyte,* which is a red blood cell.)

Demonstrate your recognition of word parts by writing answers to the following exercise. Do not be concerned if you do not recognize the meanings of the word parts, because you will learn them in subsequent chapters. After writing answers in the blanks, check your answers with the solutions found in the back of the book. It is best to work all of a particular exercise before checking your answers. It is also important to confirm your answers before going on to the next exercise. (If you have made a mistake, you do not want to keep repeating it throughout the chapter!)

EXERCISE I

Write the correct answer in each blank space.

1. Which is a combining form, cyst or cyst/o? _____
2. In chlor/o/plast, _____ is the combining form.
3. Of the following word parts, hepat/o, -algia, an-, -ase, supra-, -ose, which are prefixes? _____ and _____
4. Using the same list of word parts presented in question 3, which of the word parts are suffixes? _____, _____, and _____
5. Which type of word part (word root, prefix, or suffix) is -cyte? _____
6. Which type of word part (word root, prefix, or suffix) is de-? _____

(Check your answers with the solutions in the back of the book.)

COMBINING WORD PARTS TO WRITE MEDICAL TERMS

Remember that when combining forms are written alone, they contain a combining vowel, usually an *o*, as in hepat/o. When writing medical terms, the vowel at the end of a combining form is not always used. The following rule will help you in writing medical terms:

The combining vowel is used before suffixes that begin with a consonant and before another word root. In other words, drop the combining vowel if the suffix also begins with a vowel (a, e, i, o, or u).

 Example 1: When the comining form hepat/o is joined with the suffix -megaly, the combining vowel is used and results in the term hepatomegaly. Notice that -megaly begins with a consonant (hepat/o + -megaly = hepatomegaly).
 Example 2: When the combining form hepat/o is joined with the suffix -itis, the combining vowel is **not** used and results in the term hepatitis. Notice that the o is dropped from hepat/o because -itis begins with a vowel (hepat/o + -itis = hepatitis).
 There are exceptions to this rule in regard to use of the combining vowel, and you will learn these exceptions as you progress through the material.
 Most prefixes end with a vowel and may be added to other word parts without change. For example, precancer, preeruptive, and pre-operative result when the prefix *pre-* is joined with cancer, eruptive, and operative.

There are exceptions to the rule concerning the use of prefixes to write words. These exceptions will be noted when they occur. One exception is anti-. When anti- is joined with biotic and coagulant, the terms antibiotic and anticoagulant result. Often, however, ant- is used when the prefix is joined to a vowel. The term antacid results when ant- is joined with acid.

Sometimes two terms are acceptable when a prefix is used to form a new word. End- and endo- both mean inside. The former is usually joined with word parts beginning with a vowel, as in the term endarterial (end- + arterial). Common usage, however, has determined whether end- or endo- is used in certain cases. Some terms accept either prefix, as in endaortitis and endoaortitis. Both terms are acceptable and have identical meanings.

Demonstrate your understanding of the rules for combining word parts by working the following exercise. Do not be concerned about exceptions to the rules in this exercise.

EXERCISE II

Write the correct answer in each blank space.

1. Practice the rule for combining word parts by writing a word using appendic/o and -itis: _____
2. Write a term by joining enter/o and -al: _____
3. Join anti- and anxiety: _____
4. Join anti- and septic: _____
5. Write a word using leuk/o and -cyte: _____
6. Which type of word part is hyper-? _____
7. Combine hyper- and -emia: _____
8. Combine end- and arterectomy: _____
9. Combine endo- and cardi/o and -al: _____
10. Combine esophag/o and gastr/o and -stomy: _____

(Check your answers. If your answers are correct, you understand basic word parts and the rules for joining them to form medical terms. If your answers are incorrect, you need to read Chapter 1 again and be sure that you understand the material before proceeding to Chapter 2.)

PRONUNCIATION OF MEDICAL TERMS

In the remaining chapters in this book, pronunciation of terms will be shown in a footnote at the bottom of the page on which the term appears for the first time. Phonetic spelling is used to show pronunciation in all footnotes. This phonetic spelling uses a minimum of diacritical marks.

GUIDE TO PRONUNCIATION USED IN THIS BOOK

1. The primary (′) and secondary (″) accents are indicated.

2. An unmarked vowel ending a syllable is long. For example,
fa, pa, etc., are pronounced to rhyme with day
de, re, etc., rhyme with fee
di, pi, etc., rhyme with high
do, no, etc., rhyme with so
hu, tu, etc., rhyme with few

3. An unmarked vowel within a syllable is short. Had, bad, in, not, rug, and good are examples of words that have phonetic spellings that are the same as their usual spellings.

4. When a long vowel occurs within a syllable that must end with a consonant, the long vowel is indicated by a macron (ā, ē, ī, ō, and ū)—for example, abate (ah bāt′) and anterior (an tēr′ e or). These long vowels have the same sounds as those listed in 2, above.

5. A short vowel alone or ending a syllable is indicated by the use of the breve (ă, ĕ, ĭ, ŏ, and ŭ)—for example, catheter (kath′ ĕ ter) and coronary (kor′ ŏ na re). These short vowels have the same sound as the short vowels listed in 3, above.

Pronunciation of most medical terms follows the same rules that govern the pronunciation of all English words. Some general rules and examples that will assist you in pronunciation are given below. Remember that there are exceptions to these rules, and certain terms can have more than one acceptable pronunciation. Also, different pronunciations are often found in different parts of the United States. The pronunciations shown in this book are those recommended by *Dorland's Medical Dictionary* (W. B. Saunders Company) and *Taber's Cyclopedic Medical Dictionary* (F. A. Davis Company). Diseases, disorders, and procedures sometimes incorporate proper names, however, which may be exceptions to English pronunciation.

BASIC RULES FOR PRONUNCIATION

- c and g have the soft sounds of s and j, respectively, before e, i, and y (e.g., center, circulation, cytoplasm, generic, ginger, gymnastics. There are exceptions, and sometimes more than one pronunciation is acceptable. Gynecology is pronounced as gi or jin, using either the soft or hard g sound.)
- c and g have hard sounds before a, o, and u (e.g., cardiac, cone, cure, gas, gonorrhea, gum).

BASIC RULES FOR PRONUNCIATION (Continued)

- ch is sometimes pronounced like k (e.g., chronic, chemical).
- k has a hard sound except when occurring as kn (e.g., leukocyte and kidney have hard sounds, but k is not pronounced in knee).
- pn is pronounced as n (e.g., pneumonia).
- ps is pronounced as s (e.g., psychiatry).
- ae at the end of a word is pronounced as a long e (e.g., the plural form of patella is patellae and is pronounced pah tel' e).
- i at the end of a word is pronounced as a long i (e.g., fungi is fun ji).

2

Using Suffixes and Combining Forms to Write Medical Terms

OBJECTIVES

After completing Chapter 2, you will be able to

1. Write the meanings of the suffixes and combining forms presented in this chapter or choose their correct meaning when presented with several answers.
2. Combine word roots and suffixes correctly to form medical terms.
3. Analyze all terms studied in this chapter and demonstrate comprehension either by writing the term when presented with its definition or by selecting the correct meaning of the term from several answers.

OUTLINE

HOW SUFFIXES ARE USED TO WRITE WORDS
SUFFIXES THAT PERTAIN TO SURGICAL PROCEDURES
COMBINING FORMS
SUFFIXES THAT PERTAIN TO SYMPTOMS AND DIAGNOSIS
ADDITIONAL SUFFIXES
ADDITIONAL COMBINING FORMS
COMPREHENSIVE REVIEW EXERCISES

**HOW SUFFIXES
ARE USED TO
WRITE WORDS**

**Suffixes form nouns, adjectives, and verbs when combined with
other word parts. When a suffix that begins with a vowel is
joined with a combining form, the combining vowel is almost
always dropped from the combining form.**

Some students find it helpful to know what types of words are formed
by the use of various suffixes. It is for these students that this information about word usage is provided.

It is logical that a suffix coincides with how its meaning is used
in speech. For example, append/ectomy means surgical removal
(-ectomy) of the appendix (append/o). Appendectomy is a surgical
procedure; thus, appendectomy is a noun. From this we see that the
suffix -ectomy is used to write nouns.

Many suffixes will be learned in this chapter. Although suffixes
are emphasized, a limited number of combining forms are also presented. Combining forms are needed to write medical words, and
learning terms is easier and more interesting than only memorizing
suffixes. To make the suffixes easier to remember, they are divided
into the following sections: Suffixes that Pertain to Surgical Procedures, Suffixes that Pertain to Symptoms and Diagnosis, and Additional Suffixes.

**SUFFIXES THAT
PERTAIN TO
SURGICAL
PROCEDURES**

A list of suffixes pertaining to surgical procedures follows. Commit
the meaning of these suffixes to **memory.** It is necessary to take some
time now to memorize the suffixes and their meanings, and this can
be done in several ways. One way is to read each suffix, its meaning,
and its word association (a familiar word associated with the suffix).
Also think of words you may know that can help you to remember the
meaning. After you have studied the list for a few minutes and feel
that you know it, cover the column that contains the meanings and
word associations and then check to make sure that you know each
meaning. After you have memorized the list, write the answers to the
exercise that follows.

SUFFIXES THAT PERTAIN TO SURGICAL PROCEDURES

(All the suffixes in this list form nouns when combined with other word parts.)

Suffix	Meaning	Word Association
-centesis	surgical puncture to aspirate or remove fluid	*Amniocentesis*[1] is *puncture* of the amnion for removing fluid for study or administering treatment to the fetus.
-ectomy	excision (surgical removal or cutting out)	*Appendectomy*[2] is *excision* of the appendix.
-lysis	process of loosening, freeing, or destroying	This suffix is also used in nonsurgical words to mean *destruction* or dissolving, as in the word *hemolysis*.[3]
-pexy	surgical fixation (fastening in a fixed position)	*Mastopexy*[4] is plastic surgery that fastens breasts in a *fixed position* to correct sagging.
-plasty	surgical repair	*Plastic* is derived from the same word root as *-plasty*. *Plastic* surgery *repairs*, restores, and reconstructs body structures.
-rrhaphy	suture (uniting a wound by stitches)	This suffix is not generally used in everyday language.
-scopy	visual examination with a lighted instrument (this is not always a surgical procedure)	*Microscopy*[5] is *visual examination* of very small objects with a magnifying instrument.

---

[1] am″ne o sen te′sis
[2] ap″en dek′to me
[3] he mol′ĭ sis

[4] mas′to pek se
[5] mi kros′ko pe

SUFFIXES THAT PERTAIN TO SURGICAL PROCEDURES (Continued)

Suffix	Meaning	Word Association
-stomy	formation of an opening	A *tracheostomy*[6] is an operation that *forms a new opening* into the trachea (windpipe).
-tome	an instrument used for cutting	A *microtome*[7] is an *instrument used for cutting* thin sections of tissue for microscopic study.
-tomy	incision[8] (cutting into tissue)	A *tracheotomy*[9] is an *incision* of the trachea[10] through the skin and muscles in the neck that overlie the trachea (windpipe).
-tripsy	surgical crushing	*Lithotripsy*[11] is *surgical crushing* of a stone in the bladder.

EXERCISE I

Match the suffixes in the right column with their meanings in the left column.

_____ 1. formation of an opening   A. -centesis

_____ 2. incision   B. -ectomy

_____ 3. surgical repair   C. -lysis

_____ 4. an instrument used for cutting   D. -pexy

      E. -plasty

_____ 5. process of destroying   F. -rrhaphy

_____ 6. surgical puncture   G. -scopy

      H. -stomy

_____ 7. visual examination with an intrument   I. -tome

      J. -tomy

      K. -tripsy

---

[6] tra″ke os′to me

[7] mi′kro tōm

[8] in sizh′un

[9] tra″ke ot′o me

[10] tra′ke ah

[11] lith′o trip″se

____ 8. excision
____ 9. surgical fixa-
      tion
____ 10. suture
____ 11. surgical crush-
      ing (this suffix
      specifically
      means "crush-
      ing" and not
      destruction by
      any other
      means)

(Check your answers with the solutions in the back of the book.)

COMBINING FORMS

Combining forms for several body structures are presented below. This is not intended to be a complete list. Many combining forms will be presented in later chapters, which discuss major body systems. You should commit the following list to **memory** because subsequent chapters assume that you have already learned these combining forms. Practice learning the material here in the same manner as you learned the list of suffixes pertaining to surgical procedures that were presented earlier. Read the term, its meaning, and word association. When you think you know the material, cover the two columns on the right and try to recall the meaning of each combining form. These combining forms will be used with the aforementioned suffixes to study medical terminology in more detail and to learn how to build words. Read on!

COMBINING FORMS FOR SELECTED BODY STRUCTURES

Combining Form	Meaning	Word Association
aden/o	gland	*Adenoids*[12] were so named because they resembled or were thought to be *glands.*
angi/o	vessel	*Angiograms*[13] are x-ray records of the blood *vessels.*

---

[12] ad'ĕ noidz   [13] an'je o gramz"

**COMBINING FORMS
FOR SELECTED BODY
STRUCTURES**
(Continued)

Combining Form	Meaning	Word Association
append/o, appendic/o	appendix	An *appendectomy* is excision of the *appendix*.
cerebr/o, encephal/o (cerebr/o sometimes means cerebrum,[15] the main portion of the brain)	brain	*Cerebral*[14] palsy is paralysis caused by a brain defect. *Encephalitis*[16] is inflammation of the brain.
cutane/o, derm/a, dermat/o	skin	*Cutaneous*[17] means pertaining to the skin. A *dermatologist*[18] is a specialist who treats diseases of the skin.
mamm/o, mast/o	breast	*Mammography*[19] is the use of x-ray to diagnose breast diseases. *Mastectomy*[20] is surgical removal of the breast.
neur/o	nerve	A *neurosurgeon*[21] performs surgery on the nerves and nervous system. *Neurotic* is affected with a neurosis,[22] a type of nervous disorder.
ophthalm/o	eye	An *ophthalmologist*[23] is a specialist who treats diseases of the eye.
ot/o	ear	*Otitis*[24] is inflammation of the ear.

[14] ser'ĕ bral, sĕ re'bral
[15] ser'ĕ brum, sĕ re'brum
[16] en"sef ah li'tis
[17] ku ta'ne us
[18] der"mah tol'o jist
[19] mam og'rah fe

[20] mas tek'to me
[21] nu"ro sur'jun
[22] nu ro'sis
[23] of"thal mol'o jist
[24] o ti'tis

COMBINING FORMS FOR SELECTED BODY STRUCTURES (Continued)

Combining Form	Meaning	Word Association
tonsill/o	tonsil	*Tonsillitis*[25] is inflammation of the *tonsils*.
vas/o	vessel; ductus deferens[27] (also called vas deferens, excretory duct of the testicle)	*Vascular*[26] pertains to blood *vessels*. (Vascular is derived from a Latin word that means small vessel.)

Now let's use the combining forms you have learned with suffixes you learned earlier to explore some new medical terms. The learning method that you will be using in this book is known as semiprogrammed. The prefix semi- means half or partly. It is used in medical terms and in common words. Semiprogrammed study means that the programmed format will be used in some but not all the material. Programmed learning is a method that begins with what you already know and teaches new concepts by the progressive introduction of new information or ideas. In some ways it is similar to using a computer program, because it tells you immediately if you are right and allows you to learn at your own speed. The primary difference is that here you write your answers in the blanks that are provided. It is a proven effective and easy way to learn medical terminology.

PROGRAMMED LEARNING

1. You need to know certain things to use the programmed learning method effectively. Programmed learning consists of several blocks of material in which you sometimes will be asked to write answers about information that you have already been given.

2. The left column is the answer column, which needs to be covered. To do this, fold a piece of typing paper lengthwise or use the card attached to the back cover and position it so that it covers only the answer column.

3. In programmed learning, each block of information preceded by a number is called a frame. This is the third frame of this chapter.

---

[25] ton"sĭ li'tis

[26] vas'ku lar

[27] duk'tus def'er enz

Within most of the following frames there will be one or more blanks in which to write an answer. After writing your answer in the blank, check to see if it is correct by sliding the paper down so that the answer column on the left of the frame is uncovered.

frame

4. You are using the programmed learning method. A block of information with a number is called a _____. (Write an answer in the blank.) Whenever you see frames, you will recognize that you are learning by the programmed method.

two

5. Always check your answer immediately. The number of blanks indicate the number of words needed. For example, "_____ _____" requires how many words? _____

6. If your answer is incorrect, look back at previous frames to determine where you went wrong. You are now ready to put this information to use.

7. In Chapter 1 you learned how to write words using combining forms, prefixes, and suffixes. Combine ophthalm/o and -ic to write a word that means pertaining to the eye:

ophthalmic[28]

8. Be sure that you dropped the o from ophthalm/o before adding -ic. Ready for a bigger challenge? Don't worry about the meaning of these word parts now—you'll know the meaning of this word by the time you finish the book. Write a word using oophor/o plus salping/o plus hyster/o plus -ectomy: _____

**oophoro-
salpingo-
hysterectomy[29]**

9. You will learn later that col/o is the combining form for the colon (large intestine). Combine col/o plus the suffix for "formation of an opening": _____ Congratulations if you remembered the suffix and used it correctly! You can already write a limited number of medical terms and the number will increase rapidly by the use of this method.

colostomy[30]

[28] of thal'mik
[29] o of"o ro sal" pin go
his"ter ek'to me

[30] ko los'to me

10. Did you remember to check your answer immediately? Always be certain that you have spelled the word correctly. A colostomy is an opening of some portion of the large intestine onto the abdominal surface. This type of surgery is performed when solid waste (feces) cannot be eliminated through the normal opening because of some pathologic condition.

colo/scopy

11. In addition to writing medical terms, you will also learn how to divide words into their component parts and to analyze their meanings. We use diagonal slash marks to show the component parts of a word—for example, colo/stomy. Observe that col/o (colon) is joined to -stomy, the suffix that you just learned that means formation of an opening. When analyzing difficult terms, look for familiar word parts. Divide coloscopy[31] into its component parts: ___ ___ ___

12. Several words are usually required to state the meaning of a term. Often the definition may be stated in various ways, all equally correct. When you are asked to state something in your own words, and several words are required, this will be indicated by a long line running the width of this column—for example,

_____

**examining
the colon**

13. Knowing that colo/stomy means formation of an opening into the colon, analyze and define coloscopy:

_____

(Hint: In analyzing medical terms, it is usually helpful to begin by defining the suffix first and then to continue through the other word parts.)

**surgical fixation of
the colon**

14. Analyze the meaning of colopexy[32].

_____

Colopexy is a surgical procedure in which the colon is sutured (surgically fixed, sewn or otherwise) to the abdominal wall.

surgical fixation

15. Masto/pexy is _____ of the breast. Mastopexy corrects sagging breasts by surgical fixation. You may be wondering if mammopexy is also correct. Although it

---

[31] ko los'ko pe   [32] ko'lo pek"se

may be a word, it is not commonly used. You will learn the more commonly used terms as you progress through the material.

excision
excision

16. You learned earlier that -ectomy means ____ _____. Mastectomy is ____ of a breast. Mastectomy is sometimes performed when cancer of the breast is present, but certainly not always. The surgeon might elect to remove only the suspicious mass.

17. A breast biopsy is often done when a suspicious lump is found in the breast. A biopsy[33] is excision of a small piece of living tissue for microscopic examination, usually performed to establish a diagnosis. The biopsy can be performed with a needle (needle biopsy) or by incision of the suspicious lump. The procedure of removing a lump is sometimes called a lumpectomy. Excision of a small piece of living tissue for microscopic examination is called _____.

biopsy

18. Combine mast/o and -itis to write a word that means inflammation of the breast: _____

mastitis[34]

19. You learned that aden/o means ____. Write a word that means excision of a gland: ____ This term does not define which gland is removed, because aden/o is a general term for gland.

gland
adenectomy[35]

20. Neur/ectomy[36] is partial or total excision of a ____. (Notice that partial or total is implied. Literal translation does not always indicate the full meaning.)

nerve

21. Now write a word that means destruction of nerve tissue (or loosening of adhesions surrounding a nerve): Nice job if you knew this one! It was a little more difficult but several medical terms have more than one meaning.

neurolysis[37]

[33] bi'op se
[34] mas ti'tis
[35] ad"ĕ nek'to me
[36] nu rek'to me
[37] nu rol'ĭ sis

neurotripsy[38]

22. Now change the suffix of neuro/lysis to form a word that specifically means surgical crushing of a nerve: _____

neuroplasty[39]

23. Use a different suffix to write a word that means surgical repair of a nerve or nerves: _____

ophthalmoplasty[40]
otoplasty[41]

24. Using neuroplasty as a model, write words for the following:
surgical repair of the eye _____
surgical repair of the ear _____

skin

25. Cutane/ous means pertaining to the _____.

pertaining to

26. In the previous frame, you saw that -ous is a suffix that means _____. (Sometimes it can also mean characterized by.)

skin

27. Dermato/plasty[42] is surgical repair of the _____.
This is skin grafting or transplantation of living skin to cover defects caused by injury, surgery, or disease.

dermatome[43]
dermatotome[44]

28. Use derm/a and dermat/o to write two terms, both of which mean an instrument used to incise the skin: _____ and _____. (In anatomy dermatome has an additional meaning, but do not be concerned about its other meaning at this point.)

encephalotome[45]

29. Use encephal/o to write a word that means an instrument for incising brain tissue: _____

encephalotomy,[46]
cerebrotomy[47]

30. Write two words, both meaning incision of the brain:
_____ and _____

---

[38] nu'ro trip"se
[39] nu'ro plas"te
[40] of thal'mo plas"te
[41] o'to plas"te
[42] der'mah to plas"te

[43] der'mah tōm
[44] der'mah to tōm
[45] en sef'ah lo tōm
[46] en sef"ah lot'o me
[47] ser"ĕ brot'o me

ot/o	31. The combining form for ear is _____ , _____ .
otoplasty	32. Write a word that means surgical repair (plastic surgery of) the ear: _
ophthalmoplasty	33. Plastic surgery of the eye is _
angioplasty[48]	34. Use angi/o to write a word that means plastic surgery on vessels (blood vessels, in this case):
angiorrhaphy[49]	35. Use angio/plasty as a model to write a word that means suture of a vessel (especially a blood vessel):
angiectomy[50]	36. Use the last word you wrote as a model to form a word that means excision or cutting out of a blood vessel: _
appendectomy	37. Use append /o to write a word that means removal of the appendix: _
tonsillectomy[51]	38. Write a word that means excision of the tonsils: _
puncture	39. The amnion is the thin transparent membrane that surrounds the fetus (unborn child). Amnio/centesis is surgical _____ ____ of the amnion.
	40. See how easy it is to learn new words using the programmed method! You are already writing impressive medical terms.

SUFFIXES THAT PERTAIN TO SYMPTOMS AND DIAGNOSIS

Commit the following suffixes and their meanings to **memory.** Remember to read each suffix, its meaning, and the word association that is presented. Be certain that you are familiar with this information before proceeding to Exercise II.

---

[48] an'je o plas"te   [50] an"je ek'to me
[49] an"je or'ah fe   [51] ton"sĭ lek'to me

SUFFIXES THAT PERTAIN TO SYMPTOMS AND DIAGNOSIS

(All the suffixes listed form nouns, unless otherwise stated.)

Suffix	Meaning	Word Association
-algia	pain	Neuralgia[52] is pain along the course of a nerve.
-cele	hernia (protrusion of all or part of an organ through the wall of a cavity that contains it)	
-ectasia, -ectasis	dilatation[53] (dilation, enlargement) or stretching of a structure or part	
-edema	swelling	Edema[54] is a word that means the presence of abnormally large amounts of fluid in the tissues; it is usually applied to an accumulation of excessive fluid in the subcutaneous tissues, resulting in swelling.
-emesis	vomiting	Emesis[55] is a word that means vomiting.
-ia, -iasis	condition	Hysteria is a condition so named because hysterical women were thought to suffer from a disturbed condition of the uterus (hyster/o). Psoriasis[56] is a diseased condition of the skin marked by itchy lesions (from the Greek psora, which means itch).

---

[52] nu ral'je ah
[53] dil ah ta'shun
[54] ĕ de'mah

[55] em'ĕ sis
[56] so ri'ah sis

SUFFIXES THAT PERTAIN TO SYMPTOMS AND DIAGNOSIS (Continued)

Suffix	Meaning	Word Association
-itis	inflammation	Appendicitis[57] is inflammation of the appendix.
-malacia	soft, softening	Osteomalacia[58] is softening of the bones.
-mania	excessive preoccupation	In kleptomania[59] there is excessive preoccupation that leads to stealing things on impulse.
-megaly	enlargement	You may be more familiar with mega-. Both mega- and megal- mean large, as in megalopolis, a large city, and megaton, a large explosive force.
-oid (forms adjectives and nouns)	resembling	Mucoid[60] means similar to or resembling mucus.[61] Paranoid means resembling paranoia,[62] a psychotic disorder characterized by delusions of persecution.
-oma	tumor	Carcinoma[63] is cancer, or a cancerous tumor.
-osis	condition (often an abnormal condition; sometimes, an increase)	Neurosis is a nervous condition (disorder) that is not caused by a demonstrable structural change.

[57] ah pen″di sǐ′tis
[58] os″te o mah la′she ah
[59] klep″to ma′ne ah
[60] mu′koid
[61] mu′kus
[62] par″ah noi′ah
[63] kar″sǐ no′mah

SUFFIXES THAT PERTAIN TO SYMPTOMS AND DIAGNOSIS (Continued)

Suffix	Meaning	Word Association
-pathy	disease	The suffix -*pathy* is derived from the same source as many words that contain path/o— for example, *pathogenic*[64] organisms can cause *disease*.
-penia	deficiency	
-phobia	abnormal fear	*Hydrophobia*[65] is another term for rabies, a viral disease transmitted to humans by the bite of an infected animal. It was given the name hydrophobia after it was observed that stricken animals avoided water, as though they had a *fear* of it. Actually, rabid animals avoid water because they cannot swallow as a result of the paralysis caused by the virus.
-ptosis	prolapse (sagging)	*Ptosis*[66] is a word that means sagging. It often refers to *drooping* or *sagging* eyelids.
-rrhage, -rrhagia	excessive bleeding or hemorrhage	*Hemorrhage* is abnormal internal or external *bleeding*.
-rrhea	flow or discharge	A urethral[67] or vaginal[68] *discharge* is a primary feature of *gonorrhea.*[69]

---

[64] path o jen'ik
[65] hi"dro fo'be ah
[66] to'sis

[67] u re'thral
[68] vag'ĭ nal
[69] gon"o re'ah

SUFFIXES THAT PERTAIN TO SYMPTOMS AND DIAGNOSIS (Continued)

Suffix	Meaning	Word Association
-rrhexis	rupture	Translated literally, cardiorrhexis[70] means *ruptured* heart. One might think of a lover's broken heart, but cardiorrhexis is a pathologic condition in which the heart ruptures.
-spasm	twitching, cramp	Spasm[71] is a word that means involuntary and sudden movement or convulsive muscular contraction.
-stasis	stopping, controlling	Stasis[72] is a word that means slowing or *stopping.*

If you have not already done so, cover all the information in the preceding list, except the left column, which contains the suffixes. Test yourself to be certain that you recall the meaning of each suffix listed.

EXERCISE II

Match the suffixes in the right column with their meanings in the left column.

_____ 1. condition   A. -algia
_____ 2. inflammation   B. -cele
_____ 3. vomiting   C. -ectasis
_____ 4. hernia   D. -emesis
_____ 5. softening   E. -iasis
_____ 6. enlargement   F. -itis
_____ 7. pain   G. -malacia
_____ 8. dilatation   H. -mania
_____ 9. excessive   I. -megaly
      preoccupation   J. -stasis
_____ 10. controlling

[70] kar"de o rek'sis   [72] sta'sis
[71] spazm

EXERCISE III   *Circle the correct answer to complete each sentence.*

1. The suffix that means tumor is (-oid, -oma, -osis, -rrhagia).
2. The suffix meaning disease is (-pathy, -penia, -phobia, -ptosis).
3. The suffix that means flow or discharge is (-rrhage, -rrhea, -rrhexis, -penia).
4. Several of the suffixes that you learned are also words. One suffix that means cramp or twitching and that can also stand alone as a word is (ptosis, phobia, spasm, stasis).
5. Excessive bleeding is represented by the suffix (-rrhea, -rrhage, -rrhexis, -pathy).
6. The suffix -penia means (resembling, condition, deficient, rupture).
7. The suffix -rrhexis means (resembling, rupture, preoccupation, cramp).
8. The suffix -oid means (flow, hemorrhage, resembling, condition).
9. The suffix -phobia means (abnormal fear, excessive preoccupation, deficiency, stopping).
10. The suffix -ptosis means (disease, fear, prolapse, decreased).

(Remember to check your answers.)

PROGRAMMED LEARNING

Remember to cover the answers *(left column in each frame) with the folded paper, as you did earlier in this chapter. Write an answer in each blank and then check your answer before proceeding to the next frame.*

inflammation	1. In studying the suffixes pertaining to symptoms and diagnosis, you learned that -itis means _____.
ophthalm/o **ophthalmitis**[73]	2. The combining form for eye is _____. Write a word that means inflammation of the eye: _____
appendicitis	3. Using the combining form appendic/o (meaning appendix), write a word that means inflammation of the appendix: _____ (See how easy it is to write medical terms using this method!)

[73] of"thal mi'tis

pain	4. When analyzing the term neur/algia, we see that it is derived from neur/o (meaning nerve) and the suffix -algia. Neur/algia means _____pain_____ along a nerve.
pain **eye**	5. Ophthalm/algia[74] is _____pain_____ of the _____eye_____.
hernia	6. The list of suffixes that pertain to symptoms and diagnosis contains a word meaning protrusion of all or part of an organ through the wall of a cavity that normally contains it. This word is _____cele-hernia_____
-cele	7. The suffix that means hernia is _____cele_____.
hernia (or herniation)	8. An encephalo/cele[75] is _____hernia_____ of the brain through an opening in the skull. (This is also called a cerebral hernia.)
hernia	9. Gastr/o means stomach. A gastro/cele[76] is a _____hernia_____ of the stomach.
vomiting	10. Hyper/emesis[77] means excessive _____vomiting_____. Hyper- means excessive or above normal.
vomiting	11. Hemat/emesis[78] is _____vomiting_____ of blood. Hemat/o means blood.
prolapse **prolapse**	12. Ptosis means sag or _____prolapse_____. Blepharo/ptosis[79] is _____prolapse_____ of the eyelid. Blephar/o means eyelid.
-rrhagia	13. The suffix -rrhage means excessive bleeding. The suffix for forming words to indicate hemorrhage is _____rrhagia_____.
hemorrhage	14. Ophthalmo/rrhagia[80] is _____hemorrhage_____ from the eye.

[74] of"thal mal'je ah
[75] en sef'ah lo sēl
[76] gas'tro sēl
[77] hi"per em'ĕ sis

[78] hem"ah tem'ĕ sis
[79] blef"ah ro to'sis
[80] of thal"mo ra'je ah

discharge

15. Another suffix beginning with a double r is -rrhea. In the sexually transmitted disease gono/rrhea, -rrhea refers to the heavy _discharge_ that is characteristic of the disease.

rupture

16. You may already be familiar with the term "cardiologist,"[81] which means a physician who specializes in diseases of the heart. Cardi/o means heart. Cardio/rrhexis is _rupture_ of the heart.

ophthalmorrhexis[82]

17. Using ophthalm/o and the suffix for rupture, write a word that means rupture of the eyeball: _ophthalmorrhexis_ Translated literally, the word means rupture of the eye.

chirospasm[83]

18. Chir/o means hand. The word that means cramping of the hand is _chirospasm_. This is sometimes called writer's cramp.

angiectasia[84]
angiectasis[85]

19. Using angi/o write two words, either of which means dilation of a blood or lymph vessel: _angiectasia_ or _angiectasis_

softening

20. Osteo/malacia is a disease marked by increased _softening_ of the bone (oste/o means bone).

excessive preoccupation

21. You have probably heard of the word pyromaniac.[86] Pyro/mania[87] is _excessive preoccupation_ with fire. Pyromaniacs enjoy watching or setting fires (pyr/o means fire).

pyrophobia[88]

22. Add another suffix to pyr/o to form a word that means abnormal fear of fire: _pyrophobia_

enlargement

23. Cardio/megaly[89] is _enlargement_ of the heart.

---

[81] kar de ol'o jist
[82] of thal"mo rek'sis
[83] ki'ro spazm
[84] an"je ek ta'ze ah
[85] an"je ek'tah sis

[86] pi"ro ma'ne ak
[87] pi"ro ma'ne ah
[88] pi"ro fo'be ah
[89] kar"de o meg'ah le

resembling	24. Muc/o means mucus. Muc/oid means _resembling_ mucus.
tumor	25. Carcinoma is a synonym for cancer. Carcin/oma is a cancerous growth or malignant _tumor_.
condition	26. The suffix -osis means condition, but it sometimes implies a disease or abnormal increase. Dermat/osis[90] is a skin _condition_. (Specifically, a dermatosis is any skin condition in which inflammation is not necessarily a symptom.)
-pathy **disease, eye**	27. Another suffix you learned that means disease is _-pathy_. Ophthalmo/pathy[91] refers to any _disease_ of the _eye_.
phlebostasis[93]	28. Perhaps you are familiar with the word phlebitis,[92] which means inflammation of a vein. Add another suffix to phleb/o to write a word that means "controlling the flow of blood in a vein by means of compression": _phlebostasis_
deficiency	29. Calci/penia[94] means a _deficiency_ of calcium in body tissues and fluids.
condition	30. Lith/o is a combining form that means stone or calculus. Lith/iasis[95] is a _condition_ in which a stone or calculus is present.

ADDITIONAL SUFFIXES

Commit the following list of suffixes and their meanings to **memory**. Some important suffixes have been omitted, but they will be presented with their associated combining forms in subsequent chapters.

---

[90] der"mah to'sis   [93] flĕ bos'tah sis
[91] of"thal mop'ah the   [94] kal"sĭ pe'ne ah
[92] flĕ bi'tis   [95] lĭ thi'ah sis

SELECTED LIST OF
ADDITIONAL SUFFIXES

Suffix	Meaning	Use in Sentence
-able, -ible	capable of, able to	adjective
-ac, -al, -an, -ar, -ary, -eal, -ic, -ive, -tic	pertaining to	adjective
-ase	enzyme	noun
-iac	one who suffers	noun
-ism	condition or theory	noun
-ist	one who	noun
-ium	membrane	noun
-logist	one who studies; specialist	noun
-opia	vision	noun
-ose	sugar	noun
-ous	pertaining to or characterized by	adjective
-y	state or condition	noun

EXERCISE IV

Write the meaning of each underlined suffix. (The answer blanks are shown as one blank, even if the the answer contains more than one word.)

1. anatom<u>ist</u> _One who_____
2. immuno<u>logist</u> _Specialist_____
3. coagul<u>ase</u> _enzyme_____
4. periph<u>eral</u> _pertaining to_____
5. gluc<u>ose</u> _sugar_____
6. parasit<u>ism</u> _condition_____
7. physiolog<u>ic</u> _pertaining to_____
8. endocard<u>ium</u> _membrane_____
9. capsul<u>ar</u> _pertaining to_____
10. coagul<u>able</u> _____

(Remember to check your answers.)

PROGRAMMED LEARNING

one who, one who studies	1. You have just learned that -ist means _one who_ _____ and that -logist means _specialist_ _one who_ _studies_. The suffixes -ist and -logist are both used to form nouns. The suffix -logist is derived from log/o, meaning knowledge or study, and from -ist, but -logist is used so frequently that it is more convenient to learn the suffix form. The suffix -logist often refers to a specialist. In medicine a specialist is a person who has advanced education and training in one area of practice, such as internal medicine, dermatology,[96] or cardiology.[97]
one who	2. An anatom/ist[98] is _one_ _who_ is skilled in anatomy.
specialist	3. A patho/logist[99] is a _specialist_ in pathology,[100] the medical specialty that studies the nature and cause of disease.
pertaining to	4. Log/o is combined with -y so often that we learn -logy as a suffix form that means the study of. Whether pathology is divided as patho/logy or patho/log/y, the meaning is the same. Patho/log/ic[101] means _pertaining_ _to_ pathology or disease. (Pathological is another term that means the same as pathologic, but pathologic is the preferred form.)
ophthalmologist	5. Remembering that ophthalm/o is the combining form for eye, write a word that means an eye specialist: _ophthalmologist_
pertaining to	6. Ophthalmic means _pertaining_ _to_ the eye.
otologist[102]	7. An ear specialist is an _otologist_.

---

[96] der"mah tol'o je
[97] kar de ol'o je
[98] ah nat'o mist
[99] pah thol'o jist

[100] pah thol'o je
[101] path o loj'ik
[102] o tol'o jist

otic[103]

8. Use ophthalm/ic as a model to write a word that means pertaining to the ear: _otic_

neurologist[104]

9. Use neur/o which means nerve, to write the name of the specialist who treats diseases of the nervous system: _neurologist_

pertaining

10. A neurologist treats neural disorders. Neur/al[105] means _pertaining to_ to the nerves or nervous system.

pertaining, skin

11. Derm/al[106] means _pertaining_ to the _skin_.

skin

12. Dermatologic[107] and dermatolog/ical both mean pertaining to (or affecting) the _skin_. (These words also mean pertaining to dermatology.)

ear

13. Ot/ic means pertaining to the _ear_.

14. Many suffixes mean pertaining to, and you will have an opportunity to practice using them as you progress through the material. You learned earlier that mamm/o means breast. Mammary[108] is an adjective that means _pertaining_ to the breast.

pertaining

15. Enzymat/ic[109] means pertaining to enzymes. The suffix that means enzyme is _ase_. By its suffix, we know that lact/ase[110] has something to do with an _enzyme_.

-ase
enzyme

16. Lact/o means milk. Lact/ase is an _enzyme_ that acts on a sugar called lactose that is present in milk. Enzymes cause chemical changes in other substances. Enzymes are usually named by adding *ase* to the combining form of the substance on which they act. (For example, the enzyme fruct/ase[111] acts on the sugar fruct/ose.)

enzyme

---

[103] o'tik
[104] nu rol'o jist
[105] nu'ral
[106] derm'al
[107] der"mah to loj'ik

[108] mam'er e
[109] en"zi mat'ik
[110] lak'tās
[111] fruk'tās

sugar
lactase

17. Remember that lact/o means milk. Translated literally, lact/ose means milk _sugar_. The enzyme that acts on lactose is called _lactase_.

lip/o
enzyme
fat

18. Lip/o means fat. Fats are also called lipids,[112] which should help you to remember the combining form for fat: _lip/o_. Lip/ase[113] is an _enzyme_ that breaks down _fat_.

amylase[114]

19. Amyl/o means starch. Write the term that means an enzyme that breaks down starch: _amylase_

-lysis
starch

20. If you remember, write the suffix for destruction? _lysis_ Amylo/lysis[115] is the destruction (digestion) of _starch_.

sugar

21. Glyc/o means sugar. Glyco/lysis[116] is the breaking down of _sugar_, which is accomplished by enzymes. These enzymes are named according to the specific sugar they act on. Fructase is an enzyme that acts on fructose, a type of sugar found in fruit. Sucrase acts on sucrose, common table sugar.

proteinase,[117]
protease[118]

22. Protein/o or prote/o means protein. Write two words, either of which means an enzyme that breaks down protein: _proteinase_ and _protease_

23. The breaking down or digestion of proteins is proteolysis. Proteins, as well as most things we eat, must be broken down chemically before they can be absorbed by the body.

EXERCISE V

Circle the correct answer to complete each sentence.

1. A word that means pertaining to the tonsils is (tonsillar, tonsillectomy, tonsillitis, tonsillotomy).

---

[112] lip'idz
[113] li'pās, lip'ās
[114] am'ĭ lās
[115] am″ĭ lol'ĭ sis

[116] gli kol'ĭ sis
[117] pro'te in ās
[118] pro'te ās

2. You learned earlier that -phobia is a suffix that means abnormal fear. A term that has no other meaning than pertaining to or concerning a phobia is (claustrophobia, hydrophobia, phobic, phobist).

3. Hemorrhage is abnormal internal or external discharge of blood. A disease marked by hemorrhage is called a (hematemesis, hemorrhagic, hemorrhoid, hemostasis) disease.

4. A microscope is an instrument that magnifies very small objects. Objects that are visible only by the use of a microscope are called (microid, micrology, microscopic, microscopist) objects.

5. Coagulation means clotting. The word that means capable of being coagulated is (coagulable, coagulase, coagulate, coagulant).

ADDITIONAL COMBINING FORMS

You have learned several additional combining forms in this chapter. If you do not recognize their meanings in the following list, commit them to **memory** before proceeding.

SELECTED COMBINING FORMS

Combining Form	Meaning	Word Association
amyl/o	starch	
blephar/o	eyelid	
cardi/o	heart	A *cardiac*[119] arrest is a *heart* attack.
chir/o	hand	
glyc/o	sugar	In *hypoglycemia*[120] the blood *sugar* level is too low.
lact/o	milk	*Milk* is secreted by a woman during *lactation*.
lip/o	fat	*Lipids* are *fats* or fatlike substances.
lith/o	stone	
muc/o	mucus	Generally, *mucous* membranes secrete *mucus*.

---

[119] kar′de ak   [120] hi″po gli se′me ah

SELECTED COMBINING FORMS (Continued)

Combining Form	Meaning	Word Association
oste/o	bone	A common type of arthritis of older persons is osteo-arthritis,[121] which involves both *bones* and joints.
prote/o, protein/o	protein	
pyr/o	fire	*Pyromaniacs* enjoy setting *fires* or seeing *fires* burn.

Comprehensive Review Exercises

WORK THE FOLLOWING EXERCISES TO TEST YOUR UNDERSTANDING OF MATE-RIAL IN CHAPTER 2. IT IS BEST TO DO ALL THE REVIEW EXERCISES BEFORE CHECKING YOUR ANSWERS.

A. Write terms by combining the word parts.

1. hemat/o + -emesis _*hematemesis*_
2. oste/o + -malacia _*osteomalacia*_
3. carcin/o + -oma _*carcinoma*_
4. lith/o + -iasis _*lithiasis*_
5. col/o + -pexy _*colapexy*_

B. Write letters in the blanks to complete each word correctly.

1. Surgical formation of a new opening from the large intestine is colo _s t o m y_.
2. Visual examination of the colon is colo _s c o p y_.
3. Surgical puncture of the amnion is amnio _c e n t e s i s_.
4. Enlargement of the heart is cardio _m e g a l y_.
5. Hernia of the stomach is gastro _c e l e_.

---

[121] os″te o ar thri′tis

6. Rupture of the heart is cardio _ _ _ _ _ _ _ _.
7. Deficiency of calcium in the body is calci _ _ _ _ _ _ _.
8. Resembling mucus is muc _ _ _.

C. Write the meaning of the suffix in each term.

1. gonorrhea _____
2. chirospasm _____
3. pyromania _____
4. pyrophobia _____
5. phlebostasis _____
6. anatomist _____

D. Circle the correct answer to complete each sentence.

1. Surgical repair of a blood vessel is (angiorrhaphy, angiectomy, angioplasty, vasectomy).
2. An instrument used for cutting thin skin slices for grafting is a(n) (dermatoplasty, dermatome, encephalotome, encephalocele).
3. Surgical removal of a breast is (mastectomy, mastopexy, encephalotomy, mammoplasty).
4. A painful eye is (ophthalmorrhagia, ophthalmorrhexis, ophthalmitis, ophthalmalgia).
5. Dilation of a blood vessel is (angiectasis, angiospasm, neuralgia, dermatotome).
6. A word that pertains to the ear is (dermal, otic, amylase, hyperemesis).
7. Inflammation of the appendix is (appendicitis, appendectomy, appendotomy, adenectomy).
8. Of the following terms, the term that is not a disease or disorder is (dermatosis, ophthalmopathy, gonorrhea, tonsillectomy).
9. The chemical breakdown of sugar is (amylolysis, glycolysis, proteolysis, neurolysis).
10. A term that means capable of coagulation is (coagulable, coagulase, coagulate, coagulant).
11. What relationship does endocardium have to the heart? It is (a surgical procedure performed on the heart, an instrument used in heart surgery, a membrane within the heart, an instrument used to view the heart).
12. Dystrophic pertains to a disorder caused by defective nutrition or metabolism. A general name for this type of disorder is (dystonia, dystrophobia, dystrophic, dystrophy).

E. Write names of the following medical specialists:

1. eye specialist _____

2. ear specialist _____

3. specialist dealing with the nerves and nervous system

_____

F. Write a word in each blank to correctly complete the table.

Substance Acted On	Name of Enzyme
1. lipid	_____
2. protein	_____
or	_____
3. starch	_____
4. _____	lactase

G. Write the medical term for which each meaning is given:

1. surgical removal of a gland _____

2. surgical repair of the ear _____

3. surgical crushing of a nerve _____

4. any disease of the eye _____

5. excision (or resection) of a nerve _____

3

Using Prefixes, Suffixes, and Combining Forms to Write Medical Terms

OBJECTIVES

After completing Chapter 3, you will be able to

1. Write the meaning of the word parts presented in this chapter, choose their correct meanings when presented with several answers, and recognize and write the meanings of the word parts when they appear in medical terms.
2. Correctly combine word parts to write medical terms.
3. Analyze and write medical terms from this chapter that use combining forms for color.
4. Analyze and write medical terms from this chapter that use prefixes for numbers, measurement, position, and direction.
5. Write the correct term when presented with its definition or description.
6. Select the correct response for terms when presented with several answers, or write their meanings.

OUTLINE

HOW PREFIXES ARE USED TO FORM WORDS
COMBINING FORMS FOR COLORS
COMBINING FORMS AND RELATED SUFFIXES
ADDITIONAL COMBINING FORMS
PREFIXES THAT PERTAIN TO NUMBERS OR MEASUREMENT
PREFIXES THAT PERTAIN TO POSITION OR DIRECTION
ADDITIONAL PREFIXES
COMPREHENSIVE REVIEW EXERCISES

HOW PREFIXES ARE USED TO FORM WORDS

Prefixes will be emphasized in this chapter, but several new combining forms and suffixes will also be introduced.

Instead of only memorizing lists of prefixes, you will learn to combine them with other word parts. Learning new terms will help you to remember the prefixes that are presented. Combining forms will be presented in three groups. You will study them as combining forms that pertain to colors, as combining forms that have the same root as several commonly used suffixes, and in a list of additional combining forms.

A prefix is placed before a word to modify its meaning. Most prefixes, including those ending with a vowel, can be added to the remainder of the word without change. Exceptions will be noted. Prefixes will be grouped as those pertaining to number or measurement, those pertaining to position or direction, and in a list of additional prefixes.

COMBINING FORMS FOR COLORS

Commit combining forms and their meanings in the following list to **memory**. Word association (familiar words derived from the same root) is included to facilitate learning the word parts.

COMBINING FORMS FOR COLORS

Combining Form	Meaning	Word Association
alb/o, leuc/o, leuk/o	white	An *albino*[1] is an individual with congenital absence of pigment in the skin, hair, and eyes. The skin and hair appear *white* because of lack of pigment. *Leukemia*[2] is a malignant disease of the blood-forming organs characterized by a marked increase in the number, as well as immature forms, of *white* blood cells, called *leukocytes*.[3]

---

[1] al bi'no
[2] loo ke'me ah

[3] loo'ko sītz

**COMBINING FORMS
FOR COLORS
(Continued)**

Combining Form	Meaning	Word Association
chlor/o	green	*Chlorophyll* is the green pigment contained in *chloroplasts* in the leaves of plants, and is the reason that plants are *green*.
cyan/o	blue	Deficiency of oxygen in the blood can cause a condition called *cyanosis*,[4] a slightly *bluish*, slatelike discoloration of the skin.
erythr/o	red	*Erythrocytes*[5] are red blood cells.
melan/o	black	A *melancholy*[6] person is sad. In ancient times, people thought the bodies of melancholy persons produced a *black* bile that caused sadness.
xanth/o	yellow	*Xanthophyll* is a *yellow* pigment in plants.

EXERCISE I

Write the meaning of each underlined word part in the blank spaces.

1. erythrocytosis[7] _____ ; _____
2. xanthosis[8] _____ ; _____
3. melanoma[9] _____ ; _____
4. leukoderma[10] _____ ; _____
5. chloropia[11] _____ ; _____

---

[4] si"ah no'sis
[5] ĕ rith'ro sītz
[6] mel'an ko le
[7] ĕ rith'ro si to'sis

[8] zan tho'sis
[9] mel"ah no'mah
[10] loo"ko der'mah
[11] klo ro'pe ah

6. albinism[12] _____ white _____ ; _condition or_
7. cyanotic[13] _____ blue _____ ; _pertaining to_

(Check your answers with the solutions in the back of the book.)

COMBINING FORMS AND RELATED SUFFIXES

Several combining forms have related suffixes that are frequently used in writing medical terms. Commit the following list to **memory.** All these suffixes are used to form nouns, with the exception of those ending in -ic. (The suffixes -genic, -lytic, -phagic, and -trophic are used to form adjectives, words that modify or describe nouns. The suffix -ic can also be used to form words with several of the combining forms presented.)

SELECTED COMBINING FORMS AND RELATED SUFFIXES

Combining Form	Meaning	Suffixes
gen/o	beginning, origin	
	produced by or in	-genic
	producing or forming	-genesis
gram/o	to record	
	a record	-gram
	instrument for recording	-graph
	process of recording	-graphy
kinesi/o	movement	
	movement, motion	-kinesia, -kinesis
log/o	knowledge, words	
	one who studies, specialist	-logist
	study or science of	-logy
lys/o	destruction, dissolving	
	that which destroys	-lysin
	process of destroying	-lysis
	capable of destroying	-lytic (*Careful:* Note the change in s to t in the spelling of this suffix.)
malac/o	soft, softening	
	abnormal softening	-malacia

[12] al'bǐ nizm   [13] si ah not'ik

SELECTED COMBINING FORMS AND RELATED SUFFIXES (Continued)

Combining Form	Meaning	Suffixes
megal/o	large, enlarged enlargement	-megaly
metr/o	measure, uterine tissue instrument used to measure process of measuring	-meter -metry
path/o	disease	-pathy
phag/o	eat, ingest eating, swallowing	-phagia, -phagic, -phagy
phas/o	speech	-phasia
pleg/o	paralysis	-plegia
schis/o, schiz/o, schist/o	split, cleft	-schisis
scler/o	hard hardening	-sclerosis
scop/o	to examine, to view instrument used for viewing process of examining visually	-scope -scopy
troph/o	nutrition	-trophic -trophy

EXERCISE II

Write the correct answer in each blank space. Most answers require changing the suffix of a term included in the sentence.

1. An electro/cardio/gram[14] (electr/o refers to electricity and cardi/o means the heart) is a record (tracing) of the electrical impulses of the heart. The process of recording the electrical impulses of the heart is _____ and the instrument used is an _____.

2. A micro/scope[15] is an instrument for viewing small objects that

---

[14] e lek"tro kar'de o gram"   [15] mi'kro skōp

must be magnified so they can be studied. The process of viewing things with a microscope is _microscopy_.

3. Hemo/lysis[16] is the destruction of red blood cells that results in the liberation of hemoglobin, a red pigment. A substance that causes hemolysis is a _____. Hemolyze[17] is a verb that means to destroy red blood cells and cause them to release hemoglobin. Substances that cause red blood cells to hemolyze are called _____ substances, which means the same as hemolysins.[18]

4. Dermato/logy[19] is the study of skin and skin diseases. A physician who specializes in dermatology is a _dermatologist_.

5. Cephal/o means head. Cephalo/metry[20] is measurement of the dimensions of the head. A device or instrument for measuring the head is a _cephalometer_.

6. A carcino/gen[21] is a substance or agent that produces cancer. The production or origin of cancer is called _____. A _____ substance causes cancer.

7. Patho/logy[22] is the study of the changes caused by disease that affects any structure or function of the body. Ophthalmo/pathy[23] is any _disease_ of the eye.

8. Dys/trophic[24] muscle deteriorates because of defective nutrition or metabolism. Any disorder caused by defective nutrition or metabolism is called a _trophy_.

EXERCISE III

Write the meaning of each underlined word part. (The answer blanks are shown as one blank, even if the answer contains more than one word.)

Term	Meaning of Word Part
1. <u>kinesio</u>therapy[25]	movement
2. osteo<u>malacia</u>[26]	softening
3. dys<u>phagia</u>[27]	eat
4. cardio<u>megaly</u>[28]	enlargement

---

[16] he mol'ĭ sis
[17] he'mo līz
[18] he mol'ĭ sinz
[19] der mah tol'o je
[20] sef"ah lom'ĕ tre
[21] kar sin'o jen
[22] pah thol'o je

[23] of"thal mop'ah the
[24] dis trof'ik
[25] ki ne"se o ther'ah pe
[26] os"te o mah la'she ah
[27] dis fa'je ah
[28] kar"de o meg'ah le

5. arterio<u>sclerosis</u>[29]   *hardening*

6. <u>phago</u>cyte[30]   *eat*

7. <u>a</u>phasia[31]   *speech*

8. quadri<u>plegia</u>[32]   *paralysis*

9. <u>schizo</u>phrenic[33]   *split cleft*

10. dys<u>kinesia</u>[34]   *movement*

11. <u>megalo</u>cyte[35]   *enlargement*

12. rachi<u>schisis</u>[36] (spina bifida)   *split cleft*

(Check your answers.)

PROGRAMMED LEARNING

*Remember to cover the answers (left column of the frames) with
folded paper or cover card as you did in Chapter 2. Write an answer in
each blank and check your answer immediately before proceeding to
the next frame.*

	1. You already know several word parts, and we will now build on them to learn more.
large (enlarged)	2. You have learned that megal/o means *enlargement*.
large	3. A megalo/cyte is a *large* cell. (This meaning usually refers to an extremely large red blood cell.)
cell	4. You saw in the previous frame that -cyte means *cell*.
red	5. You learned earlier that erythr/o means *red*.
red cell	6. Translated literally, an erythro/cyte is a *red cell*. (This is an abbreviated way of saying red blood cell, a blood cell that carries oxygen.)

[29] ar te″re o sklĕ ro′sis
[30] fag′o sīt
[31] ah fa′ze ah
[32] kwod″ri ple′je ah

[33] skiz″o fren′ik
[34] dis″kĭ ne′ze ah
[35] meg′ah lo sīt
[36] ra kis′kĭ sis

leukocyte

7. Using erythro/cyte as a model, now use leuk/o to write a word that means white cell (or white blood cell): _leukocyte_

8. Cyt/o means cell. Combine cyt/o and the suffix that means process of visually examining to form a new word that means examination of cells: _cytoscopy_ (Congratulations if you answered this correctly. You can see that you really are learning medical terms. You might even have written a word that you've never seen before!)

cytoscopy[37]

cytology[38]

9. Write a word that means the study of cells: _cytology_

10. The combining form onc/o means tumor. Now write a word that means the study of tumors (actually the branch of medicine that deals with tumors): _oncology_

oncology[39]

11. The word tumor is used in different ways. It sometimes means a swelling or enlargement, but it often refers to a spontaneous new growth of tissue that forms an abnormal mass. This latter definition is also called a neoplasm.[40] The combining form ne/o means new. A neo/plasm is a _new_ growth of tissue that serves no useful function.

new

12. A benign[41] tumor is not cancerous, so it does not spread to other parts of the body. Malignant[42] is the opposite of benign and is descriptive of cancerous growths. A melan/oma is a malignant pigmented mole or tumor. Translated literally, a melan/oma is a _black_ tumor. Carcin/oma[43] is a synonym for cancer. The combining form carcin/o means cancer and -oma means tumor.

black

cancer

13. Carcino/gens are agents that cause _cancer_.

carcinogenesis[44]

14. Write a word that means the origin of cancer: _carcinogenesis_

---

[37] si tos'ko pe
[38] si tol'o je
[39] ong kol'o je
[40] ne'o plazm

[41] be nīn'
[42] mah lig'nant
[43] kar"sĭ no'mah
[44] kar"sĭ no jen'ĕ sis

mind	15. You are probably familiar with the term psychic,[45] a person said to be endowed with almost supernatural powers. Psych/ic also means concerning the mind, because psych/o means mind. Psychol/ogy is the science that deals with the _____ or with mental processes and their effects on behavior.
mind	16. Psycho/genic[46] means originating in the _____.
psychogenesis[47]	17. Change psycho/genic to a word that means the origin and development of the mind, or the formation of mental traits: _____
origin	18. Litho/genesis[48] is the _____ of stones, or calculi. A calculus[49] is an abnormal concretion that forms within the body, such as a kidney stone. The combining form lith/o means stone.
dissolving (or destruction)	19. Litho/lysis[50] means _____ of stones. Large amounts of water can sometimes dissolve small stones in the bladder. A commonly used surgical procedure crushes small stones using an instrument called a lithotrite[51] or, more recently, using ultrasonic energy from a source outside the body.
lithotripsy[52]	20. The word that means surgical crushing of a stone is _____. (If you don't remember the suffix, look it up in Chapter 2. This will help you remember it.)
stones	21. Lith/iasis[53] is a condition marked by the formation of _____.
sugar	22. Glyco/lysis[54] is the breaking down of sugar by an enzyme in the body. In Chapter 2 you learned that glyc/o means _____.

[45] si′kik
[46] si″ko jen′ik
[47] si″ko jen′ĕ sis
[48] lith″o jen′ĕ sis
[49] kal′ku lus

[50] lĭ thol′ĭ sis
[51] lith′o trīt
[52] lith′o trip″se
[53] lĭ thi′ah sis
[54] gli kol′ĭ sis

23. Most sugars that we consume are converted to glyco/gen[55] and stored for future conversion into glucose, which is used for performing work. Sugars and starches (carbohydrates) are important in providing the body with energy. Glucose is the most important carbohydrate in metabolism because cells use glucose for energy.

fat
fat (fatty)

24. Lipids are fats that are used by our bodies to store energy on a long-term basis. Fats also act as insulation against cold. You learned previously that lip/o means _____ *Fat* _____. A lip/oma[56] is a benign tumor composed of _____ *Fat* _____ tissue.

destruction

25. Remembering that -lysis means dissolving or destruction, electro/lysis[57] is _____ *dissolving destruction* _____ using a electric current. Electrolysis is sometimes used to remove unwanted hair.

electroencephalography[59]

26. The combining form electr/o means electricity. An electro/encephalo/gram[58] is a record produced by the electrical impulses of the brain. The process of recording the electrical impulses of the brain is _____ *electroencephalography* _____ (That's quite an impressive word that you have written. It's abbreviated EEG.)

electroencephalograph[60]

27. Now write the name of the instrument used in electroencephalography: _____ *electroencephalograph* _____

cephalometer[61]

28. We know that encephal/o means brain. The word is derived from en- (meaning inside) and cephal/o (meaning head). Cephalometry is measurement of the head. Change the suffix to write a word that means an instrument used to measure the head: _____ *Cephalometer* _____

29. The combining form phot/o means light. Photo/graphy is the process of making images on sensitized material (film) by exposure to light or other radiant energy. What we call a photograph is

---

[55] gli′ko jen
[56] lǐ po′mah
[57] e″lek trol′ǐ sis
[58] e lek″tro en sef′ah lo gram

[59] e lek″tro en sef″ah log′rah fe
[60] e lek″tro en sef′ah lo graf″
[61] sef″ah lom′ĕ ter

actually a "photogram," but the picture is called a photograph through common usage.

light	30. Translated literally, photo/phobia[62] is abnormal fear of ___*light*___. It means unusual sensitivity of the eyes to light. Photophobia is a common complaint of someone with German measles.
fear	31. Necro/phobia[63] is abnormal ___*fear*___ of death or dead bodies. You can see from the word necro/phobia that necr/o is a combining form meaning dead or death.
dead	32. Translated literally, necr/osis[64] means a ___*dead*___ condition. Necrosis is the death of areas of tissue or bone surrounded by healthy tissue. Necrotic tissue is dead tissue.
fire	33. Pyro/phobia is abnormal fear of fire. You can see from the term pyro/phobia that pyr/o means ___*fire*___.
fire	34. Pyro/mania[65] is abnormal preoccupation with ___*fire*___. A pyromaniac derives pleasure from seeing or setting fires.
fever	35. A pyro/gen[66] is any substance that produces fever. In this new term the meaning is implied. In an infection pyrogenic[67] bacteria produce or cause ___*fever*___ in their host, the individual who is harboring the bacteria. Pyrogenic means producing fever.
producing	36. Using pyro/genic as a model, pyo/genic[68] means ___*producing*___ pus.
pus	37. The combining form py/o means pus. Pyo/genesis[69] is the formation of ___*pus*___.

---

[62] fo"to fo'be ah
[63] nek"ro fo'be ah
[64] nĕ kro'sis
[65] pi"ro ma'ne ah

[66] pi'ro jen
[67] pi"ro jen'ik
[68] pi"o jen'ik
[69] pi"o jen'ĕ sis

pus	38. Pyo/derma[70] is any acute, inflammatory disease of the skin in which _____ is produced.
inflammation	39. Dermat/itis[71] is _____ of the skin. One type is caused by allergies, and is called allergic dermatitis.
dermatologist[72]	40. The type of physician who specializes in the treatment of skin diseases is a _____.
gerontology[74]	41. A geronto/logist[73] specializes in the treatment of elderly persons. The name of this medical specialty is _____, also known as ger/iatrics.[75] The combining forms geront/o and ger/o both refer to aged or elderly.
study	42. Histo/logy[76] is the _____ of the structure, function, and composition of tissues. The combining form hist/o means tissue.
histologist[77]	43. Write a word that means one who specializes in histology: _____
tissue	44. Histo/logic[78] pertains to _____
tissue	45. Histo/logic compatibility refers to _____ that is suitable for transplantation to another individual.
study	46. Esthesio/logy[79] is the _____ of feeling or sensory phenomena. The combining form esthesi/o means feeling or nervous sensation.
	47. In general, medicine is more concerned with an/esthesio/logy,[80] which is the science of an/esthesia[81] (an- means not or without).

---

[70] pi"o der'mah	[76] his tol'o je
[71] der"mah ti'tis	[77] his tol'o jist
[72] der"mah tol'o jist	[78] his to loj'ik
[73] jer"on tol'o jist	[79] es the"ze ol'o je
[74] jer"on tol'o je	[80] an"es the"ze ol'o je
[75] jer"e at'riks	[81] an"es the'ze ah

feeling (sensation)	An/esthes/ia means partial or complete loss of ___feeling___, with or without loss of consciousness.
sensation	48. Anesthetic[82] pertains to anesthesia. It also means the agent that produces an/esthesia, or loss of ___sensation___. Anesthetics are classified as local or general according to their action. Local anesthetics affect a local area only, rather than the entire body. General anesthetics act on the brain and cause loss of consciousness.
	49. Some people mistakenly associate anesthesia with normal sleep. A sleeping person can be awakened and normal awareness can be immediately restored, unlike someone who has been given an anesthetic.
sleep	50. The combining form narc/o means sleep. A narco/tic produces stupor or ___sleep___. A narcotic is a drug that in a moderate dose depresses the central nervous system and produces sleep. An excessive dose produces unconsciousness, stupor, coma, and possibly death.
sleep **sleep**	51. The combining form nar/co means ___sleep___. Narco/lepsy[83] is a chronic ailment that consists of recurrent attacks of drowsiness and ___sleep___.
seizure	52. The suffix -lepsy means seizure. You probably have heard of epi/lepsy,[84] a brain disorder characterized by sudden, brief attacks of altered consciousness, motor activity, or sensory phenomena. Convulsive seizures are the most common form of these attacks, and this is the basis for the naming of epilepsy. The suffix -lepsy means ___seizure___.
narcolepsy	53. Sleep seizure is another name for ___narcolepsy___ (combining form for sleep + suffix for seizure).

---

[82] an"es thet'ik
[83] nar'ko lep"se

[84] ep ĭ lep'se

thirst	54. The combining form dip/so means thirst. Poly/dips/ia[85] is a condition characterized by excessive _____ *thirst* _____ .
dips/o	55. Write the combining form that means thirst: ___ *dips/o* ___

EXERCISE IV

You have learned several combining forms as well as the prefix an- (meaning no, not, or without) and two suffixes, -cyte (meaning cell) and -lepsy (meaning seizure). The combining forms are listed in the left column. Words that correspond to the combining forms are listed alphabetically in the right column. In each blank space, write the appropriate word that corresponds to the meaning of the given combining form.

Combining Form	Meaning	Word List
1. carcin/o	*cancer*	cancer
2. cardi/o	*heart*	cell
3. cephal/o	*cephalic*	dead
4. cyt/o	*cell*	elderly
5. dips/o	*thirst*	electricity
6. electr/o	*electricity*	feeling
7. esthesi/o	*feeling*	fire
8. ger/o, geront/o	*elderly*	head
9. hist/o	*tissue*	heart
10. leps/o	*seizure*	light
11. lith/o	*stone*	mind
12. narc/o	*sleep*	new
13. necr/o	*dead*	pus
14. ne/o	*new*	seizure
15. onc/o	*tumor*	sleep
16. phot/o	*light*	stone
17. psych/o	*mind*	thirst
18. py/o	*pus*	tissue
19. pyr/o	*fire*	tumor

(*Check your answers.*)

ADDITIONAL COMBINING FORMS

Commit the following list to **memory:**

---

[85] pol"e dip'se ah

ADDITIONAL COMBINING FORMS

Combining Form	Meaning	Word Association
aer/o	air	*Aeroplane* is the British spelling of *airplane.*
blast/o	embryonic[86] form	In studying the development of organisms, the names of early (embryonic) forms have *-blast* endings. For example, embryonic bone cells are *osteoblasts.*[87]
cry/o	cold	*Cryotherapy*[88] uses *cold* temperatures to treat certain conditions.
crypt/o	hidden	A *cryptic* remark has a *hidden* meaning. A *cryptogram* is a message written in code, so it has a *hidden* meaning.
fibr/o	fiber	*Fibrous*[89] means containing, consisting of, or resembling *fiber.*
myc/o	fungus	*Mycology*[90] is a branch of botany that deals with *fungi*[91] (plural of *fungus*).
optic/o, opt/o	vision	*Optical* pertains to *vision*. An *optometrist*[92] examines the eye to determine *vision* and prescribes corrective lens, if necessary.

---

[86] em″bre on′ik
[87] os′te o blast″
[88] kri″o ther′ah pe
[89] fi′brus

[90] mi kol′o je
[91] fun′ji
[92] op tom′ĕ trist

ADDITIONAL COMBINING FORMS (Continued)

Combining Form	Meaning	Word Association
orth/o	straight, straighten	An *orthodontist*[93] is a dentist who *straightens* teeth.
pharmac/o	drugs, medicine	*Medicines* are dispensed at a *pharmacy*.
phon/o	voice	We hear someone's *voice* when we speak with them by *phone*.
therm/o	heat	*Thermal* clothing is designed to prevent loss of body *heat*.
top/o	position, place	*Topography* is often concerned with the making of maps or charts of a particular *place* or region.

EXERCISE V

You have just learned several new combining forms. Complete the following sentences by writing words in the blanks that correspond to underlined word parts.

1. A/<u>phon</u>/ia[94] is absence or loss of ___voice___ (a- means absent).
2. In an ec/<u>top</u>/ic[95] pregnancy, the embryo is implanted outside the uterus. In other words, the embryo is implanted outside the usual ___position, place___.
3. <u>Cryo</u>/surgery[96] is the destruction of tissue by application of extreme ___cold___.
4. <u>Ortho</u>/pnea[97] is a condition in which breathing is possible only when the person is sitting in an upright, or ___straight___, position (-pnea refers to breathing).
5. <u>Pharmaco</u>/therapy[98] is the treatment of disease with ___drugs___. medicine

---

[93] or"tho don'tist
[94] a fo'ne ah
[95] ek top'ik

[96] kri"o sur'jer e
[97] or"thop ne'ah
[98] fahr"mah ko ther'ah pe

6. An optic/ian[99] specializes in the translation, filling, and adapting of prescriptions, products, and accessories for _____.

7. Hyper/therm/ia[100] is a serious condition in which the body temperature is greatly elevated because of retention of body _____.

8. An aero/sol[101] is a suspension of fine particles in _____ or a gas.

9. An erythro/blast[102] is an _____ of a red blood cell.

10. Crypt/orchidism[103] is a developmental defect in which the testicles remain in the abdominal cavity. Because the testicles cannot be seen, they might be considered _____ — thus, the name cryptorchidism.

11. A fibro/lysin[104] is a substance that dissolves _____ or fibrous material.

12. Myco/dermat/itis[105] is inflammation of the skin caused by a _____.

(*Check your answers.*)

PREFIXES THAT PERTAIN TO NUMBERS OR MEASUREMENT

Many of the prefixes in the following list are used in everyday language. Common words are given to help you associate prefixes with their meanings. Commit their meanings to **memory**.

SELECTED PREFIXES THAT PERTAIN TO NUMBERS OR MEASUREMENT

Prefix	Meaning	Word Association
nulli-	none	The word *null* means having *no* value, amounting to *nothing*, or equal to *zero*.
primi-	first	*Primary* means standing *first* in rank or importance.

---

[99] op tish'an
[100] hi"per ther'me ah
[101] ār'o sol
[102] ĕ rith'ro blast

[103] krip tor'kĭ dizm
[104] fi brol'is in
[105] mi"ko der"mah ti'tis

SELECTED PREFIXES THAT PERTAIN TO NUMBERS OR MEASUREMENT (Continued)

Prefix	Meaning	Word Association
		Primitive humans were some of the *first* people on earth.
mono-, uni-	one	A *monorail* is a *single* rail that serves as a track for a wheeled vehicle. A *monocular* scope has *one* eyepiece. A *unicorn* and a *unicycle* have *one* horn and *one* wheel, respectively.
bi-, di-	two	A *bicycle* has *two* wheels. Carbon *dioxide* contains *two* atoms of oxygen.
tri-	three	A *tricycle* has *three* wheels.
quad-, quadri- tetra-	four	*Quadruplets* are *four* offspring born at one birth. A *quadriplegic*[106] is one who has paralysis of all *four* extremities (the arms and legs). A *tetrahedron* is a solid figure having *four* faces.
hemi-, semi-	half, partly	Each of the earth's *hemispheres* represents *half* of the earth. A *semicircle* is *half* of a circle.
multi-, poly-	many	A *multitude* represents *many* or several. *Multipurpose* means serving *many* purposes. *Polyunsaturated* fats have *many*

---

[106] kwod″rĭ ple′jik

SELECTED PREFIXES THAT PERTAIN TO NUMBERS OR MEASUREMENT (Continued)

Prefix	Meaning	Word Association
		unsaturated chemical bonds. *Polysaccharides*[107] are complex carbohydrates, generally composed of many molecules of simpler sugars.
hyper-	excessive, more than normal	*Hyperactive* means *excessively* active. *Hyperglycemia*[108] means an *above normal* amount of sugar in the blood.
hypo-	beneath or below normal	*Hypodermic*[109] means *under* or beneath the skin. *Hypoglycemia*[110] is a condition in which there is a *below normal* amount of sugar in the blood.
macro-	large	*Macroscopic*[111] structures are *large* enough to be seen by the naked eye.
micro-	small	A *microscope* is used to view very *small* objects.

EXERCISE VI

Complete the following sentences by writing in the blanks that correspond to the underlined prefixes.

1. Unilateral[112] pertains to _____ side of the body only.

---

[107] pol″e sak′ah rīdz
[108] hi″per gli se′me ah
[109] hi″po der′mik
[110] hi″po gli se′me ah
[111] mak″ro skop′ik
[112] u″nĭ lat′er al

2. Primi/gravida[113] refers to a female who is pregnant for the _____ *first* _____ time.

3. Translated literally, hemi/plegia[114] means paralysis of _____ *half part* _____ of the body. In this case, it means one side of the body.

4. A tri/para[115] is a female who has had _____ *3* _____ successful pregnancies.

5. Bi/focal[116] means having _____ *2* _____ focal distances. In eyeglasses, the upper part of the lens is generally used for distant vision and the lower section of the lens is used for near vision.

6. A nulli/para[117] is a female who has borne _____ *no* _____ children.

7. Semi/conscious[118] is _____ *half partial* _____ aware of one's surroundings.

8. Multi/cellular[119] means composed of _____ *many* _____ cells.

9. Translated literally, poly/dipsia means _____ *many* _____ thirsts. It actually means excessive thirst.

10. Quadri/plegia is paralysis of all _____ *4* _____ extremities.

11. Mono/nuclear[120] pertains to a cell that has how many nuclei? _____ *one* _____

12. The term hypo/calcemia[121] indicates something about the amount of calcium in the blood. It means that the amount of calcium is _____ *beneath under* _____ .

13. Hyper/lipemia[122] means _____ *excessive* _____ amount of fat in the blood.

14. Translated literally, macro/cephaly[123] means _____ *large* _____ head. It actually means excessive size of the head.

15. A micro/organism[124] is a _____ *small* _____ living organism, usually microscopic, such as bacteria, rickettsiae, viruses, molds, yeasts, and protozoa.

16. Multiple sclerosis[125] is a chronic progressive disease of the central nervous system characterized by destruction of the myelin[126] sheaths of neurons[127] (nerve cells). The damaged myelin sheaths deteriorate to scleroses[128] (scler/o means hard), hardened scars,

---

[113] pri"mĭ grav'ĭ dah
[114] hem"e ple'je ah
[115] trip"ah rah
[116] bi fo'kal
[117] nuh lip'ah rah
[118] sem"e kon'shus
[119] mul"tĭ sel'u lar
[120] mon"o nu'kle ar

[121] hi"po kal se'me ah
[122] hi"per li pe'me ah
[123] mak"ro sef'ah le
[124] mi"kro or'gan izm
[125] skle ro'sis
[126] mi'e lin
[127] nu'ronz
[128] skle ro'sēz

or plaques. The disorder is called <u>multiple</u> sclerosis because of the _____ scleroses formed on the neurons.

PREFIXES THAT PERTAIN TO POSITION OR DIRECTION

Commit the meanings of the following prefixes to **memory**. Familiar words are also listed to help you remember the prefixes.

PREFIXES THAT PERTAIN TO POSITION OR DIRECTION

Prefix	Meaning	Word Association
ab-	away from	*Abduct* means to carry *away* by force or to draw *away from* a given position.
ad-	toward	In drug *addiction* (now called chemical dependency), one is drawn *toward* a habit-forming drug. In other words, one has a compulsive physiologic need for a certain drug.
ante-, pre-, pro-	before	An *anteroom* is an outer room that is generally reached *before* a more important room. *Prehistoric* pertains to the time *before* written history. A *prologue* is an introduction that comes *before* a play, literary work, or other event.
dia-	through	The *diameter* passes *through* the center of a circle.
ecto-, ex-, exo-	out, without, away from	To *export* is to carry or send *away* to another place. The skeleton of some animals, such as insects, is on the *outer*

PREFIXES THAT PERTAIN TO POSITION OR DIRECTION (Continued)

Prefix	Meaning	Word Association
		surface and is called an *exoskeleton*.
epi-	above, on	An *epitaph* is often inscribed *on* the tombstone or grave of the person buried there.
en-, endo-	inside	*Enclose* means to close up *inside* something, to hold in, or to include.
hypo-, sub-	beneath, under	A *hypodermic* injection is made just *beneath* the skin. *Submarines* are designed for *underwater* operation.
inter-	between	An *interval* is a space of time *between* events.
intra-	within	*Intracollegiate* activities are those *within* a college or engaged in by members of a college.
meso-	middle	The *mesoderm*[129] is the *middle* of the three primary germ layers of an embryo.
peri-	around	The *perimeter* is the outer boundary or the line that is drawn *around* the outside of an area.
post-	after, behind	To *postdate* is to assign a date to something *after* the date it actually occurred, such as when you

[129] mes'o derm

PREFIXES THAT PERTAIN TO POSITION OR DIRETION (Continued)

Prefix	Meaning	Word Association
		postdate a check. *Postnasal*[130] means lying or occurring *behind* the nose.
retro-	behind, backward	*Retroactive* means extending *back* to a prior time or condition. *Retrospection* means looking *backward* in time or surveying the past.
super-, supra-	above, beyond	*Supernormal* is *beyond* normal human powers. A *suprarenal*[131] gland is situated *above* each kidney.

EXERCISE VII

Write the correct answer in each blank space.

1. Tonsillar[132] means pertaining to a tonsil. Add a prefix to tonsillar to write a word that means situated around a tonsil:
   _____

2. Tracheal[133] pertains to the trachea (the windpipe). Endo/tracheal[134] means _____ the trachea.

3. Ab/ductors are muscles that make movement possible _____ _____ the midline of the body.

4. Using the word ab/ductors as a model, write the name of muscles that are responsible for drawing a limb toward the midline of the body: _____

5. Post/partum[135] refers to the time _____ childbirth, but post/esophageal[136] means _____ the esophagus.

---

[130] pōst na′zal
[131] soo″prah re′nal
[132] ton′sĭ lar
[133] tra′ke al

[134] en″do tra′ke al
[135] pōst par′tum
[136] pōst ĕ sof″ah je′al

6. Post/nasal means occurring or situated behind the nose. Meso/nasal[137] means situated in the _middle_ of the nose. Retro/nasal[138] means situated _behind_ the nose.

7. Supra/tonsillar[139] means _above_ a tonsil.

8. Ante/natal[140] and pre/natal[141] mean occurring _before_ birth.

9. Exo/genous[142] means developing or originating _outside_ the organism. Endogenous[143] means originating within the organism.

10. Glossal[144] refers to the tongue. Hypo/glossal[145] means _beneath_ the tongue (this is also called sublingual[146]). The sub- in sub/lingual means _beneath_.

11. Inter/cellular[147] means situated _between_ the cells of a structure.

12. Dia/thermy[148] is a treatment in which heat is passed _through_ body tissues.

13. En/capsulate[149] means to enclose _within_ a capsule.

14. The prefix super- in super/ficial implies _beyond_. Superficial means situated on or near the surface.

15. The epidermis[150] is the outermost layer of skin. The prefix epi- indicates that the epi/dermis lies _above_ another structure. The epidermis lies above a skin layer called the dermis.

(Check your answers.)

ADDITIONAL PREFIXES

This final list contains additional prefixes that you should commit to **memory.** Their meanings should be easy to remember, because many of them are used in everyday language.

---

[137] mes"o na'zal
[138] ret"ro na'zal
[139] soo"prah ton'si lar
[140] an"te na'tal
[141] pre na'tal
[142] eks oj'ĕ nus
[143] en doj'ĕ nus

[144] glos'al
[145] hi"po glos'al
[146] sub ling'gwal
[147] in"ter sel'u lar
[148] di'ah ther"me
[149] en kap'su lāt
[150] ep"ĭ der'mis

A SELECTED LIST OF ADDITIONAL PREFIXES

Prefix	Meaning	Word Association
a-, an-	no, not, without	(*Rule:* Use a- before a consonant. Use an- before a vowel or the letter h.) *Asymptomatic*[151] means *without symptoms. Anesthesia* means *without feeling.*
anti-, contra-	against	An *antiperspirant* acts *against* excessive perspiration. A *contraceptive* acts *against* or prevents pregnancy. (The i in anti- is sometimes dropped before a vowel.)
brady-	slow	
dys-	bad, difficult	Reading is very *difficult* when one has *dyslexia.*[152] This disorder is thought to be an inability to organize graphic symbols.
eu-	good, normal	*Euthanasia*[153] is mercy killing and is thought by some people to be a *good* or painless death when a person is hopelessly ill.
in-	not	*Inconsistent* means *not* consistent.
mal-	bad	*Maladjusted* means poorly *(badly)* adjusted.

[151] a"simp"to mat'ik
[152] dis lek'se ah
[153] u"thah na'zhe ah

A SELECTED LIST OF ADDITIONAL PREFIXES (Continued)

Prefix	Meaning	Word Association
para-	near, beside, or abnormal	Two *parallel* lines run *beside* each other.
per-	through or by	To *perspire* is to excrete fluid *through* the pores of the skin.
tachy-	fast	A *tachometer* measures how *fast* something rotates.

EXERCISE VIII

Match the prefixes in the left column with their meanings in the right column (the choices on the right may be used more than once).

____	1. dys-	A.	good, normal
____	2. tachy-	B.	bad
____	3. brady-	C.	not
____	4. para-	D.	against
____	5. anti-	E.	fast
____	6. in-	F.	slow
____	7. mal-	G.	near, beside, abnormal
____	8. a-		
____	9. contra-		
____	10. eu-		
____	11. an-		

(Check your answers.)

EXERCISE IX

Use the underlined words as clues to the prefixes that are to be written in the dashed blanks to form the correct terms.

1. Translated literally, tachycardia[154] means fast heart. It actually means an increased pulse rate (the number of heartbeats per minute). A word that means <u>slow</u> pulse is B l a d y cardia.

2. If bradyphasia[155] is slowness of speech, <u>rapid</u> speech is _ _ _ _ _phasia.

---

[154] tak″e kar′de ah   [155] brad″e fa′ze ah

3. Hypothyroidism[156] and hyperthyroidism[157] mean decreased and increased activity of the thyroid gland, respectively. <u>Normal</u> thyroid function is _⟋__⟍_thyroidism. A person with normal thyroid function is said to be euthyroid.[158]

4. Continence[159] is the ability to refrain from yielding to desire, such as sexual desire, or from the urge to defecate or urinate. The opposite of this, <u>not</u> having continence, is called _⟋__⟍_continence.

5. Poor (<u>bad</u>) absorption of nutrients is _⟋___⟍_absorption. (Dysabsorption is not a word.)

6. An _⟋__⟍_acid acts <u>against</u> acidity, especially in the digestive tract.

7. Not capable of uniting, or <u>not</u> compatible, is _⟋__⟍_compatible.

8. A <u>difficult</u> or weak voice is _⟋__⟍_phonia.

9. Any condition that renders some particular form of treatment improper (acts <u>against</u> some particular form of treatment) is a _⟋_⟍__⟍_indication.

10. Four glands that lie <u>beside</u> the thyroid are called the _⟋_⟍__⟍_thyroid glands.

11. An _⟋_⟍__⟍_convulsive is an agent that suppresses (acts <u>against</u>) convulsions.

12. <u>Difficulty</u> in eating is _⟋__⟍_phagia.

13. Inflammation of tissue adjacent to or <u>near</u> the appendix is _⟋_⟍__⟍_appendicitis.

14. A word that literally means <u>through</u> the skin is _⟋___⟍_cutaneous.

15. The <u>para</u>thyroids are small glands that lie _⟋__⟍__⟍_the thyroid gland (sometimes embedded within the gland).

16. Hyposecretion and <u>hyper</u>secretion of the parathyroids are called hypoparathyroidism[160] and _ _ _ _ _parathyroidism, respectively.

EXERCISE X

Five terms are defined here. Form a term that means the opposite by writing a- or an- in each blank space.

1. Aerobic[161] means living only in the presence of oxygen; able to live without oxygen is _____aerobic.

---

[156] hi″po thi′roi dizm
[157] hi″per thi′roi dizm
[158] u thi′roid

[159] kon′tĭ nens
[160] hi″po par″ah thi′roid izm
[161] a er o′bik, ă ro′bik

2. Esthesia means feeling or sensation; partial or complete loss of sensation is _____esthesia.
3. Febrile[162] pertains to a fever; without fever is _____febrile.
4. Hydrous means containing water; without or lacking water is _____hydrous.
5. Symptomatic[163] means of the nature of a symptom or concerning a symptom; without symptoms is _____symptomatic.

Comprehensive Review Exercises

A. Match the underlined prefixes in the left column with their meanings in the right column (not all selections will be used).

____	1. <u>bi</u>focal	A.	none
____	2. <u>nulli</u>para	B.	one
____	3. <u>primi</u>gravida	C.	two
____	4. <u>tri</u>para	D.	three
____	5. <u>uni</u>lateral	E.	four
		G.	many
		H.	first

B. Write the meaning of each underlined prefix in the blank space.

1. <u>hypo</u>calcemia _____
2. <u>endo</u>tracheal _____
3. <u>ante</u>natal _____
4. <u>post</u>esophageal _____
5. <u>hypo</u>glossal _____
6. <u>in</u>continence _____
7. <u>tachy</u>cardia _____
8. <u>post</u>partum _____
9. <u>sub</u>lingual _____
10. <u>epi</u>dermis _____
11. <u>pre</u>natal _____
12. <u>super</u>ficial _____

---

[162] feb'ril   [163] simp"to mat'ik

C. Match the underlined word parts in the left column with their meanings in the right column (not all selections will be used and some may be used more than once).

_____	1. osteo<u>malacia</u>	A.	enlarged or large
_____	2. cardio<u>megaly</u>	B.	hardening
_____	3. arterio<u>sclerosis</u>	C.	hidden
_____	4. rachi<u>schisis</u>	D.	more than normal
_____	5. onco<u>logy</u>	E.	science of
_____	6. <u>orth</u>opnea	F.	small
_____	7. <u>crypt</u>orchidism	G.	softening
_____	8. <u>hyper</u>glycemia	H.	specialist
_____	9. <u>macro</u>scopic	I.	split
_____	10. <u>schizo</u>phrenia	J.	straight

D. Use one of the following words to correctly complete the sentences.

cephalometer   electrocardiogram   hemolysin
cephalometry   electrocardiograph   hemolysis
                 electrocardiography   hemolytic
                                         hemolyze

An (1) _____ is an instrument that records the electrical activity of the heart, and the record produced is called

an (2) _____. The name of this process is

(3) _____.

The destruction of red blood cells is called

(4) _____. A substance that causes this destruction is

a (5) _____ substance, or a (6) _____.

Measurement of the head is (7) _____ and the

instrument used is a (8) _____.

E. Circle the correct answer to complete each sentence.

1. Within a cell is (extracellular, intercellular, intracellular, multicellular).
2. Normal thyroid activity is (euthyroidism, hypothyroidism, hyperthyroidism, parathyroidism).
3. Any condition that renders a particular form of treatment undesirable is a(n) (anticonvulsive, antacid, contraindication, malabsorption).

4. A weak voice is (dysphagia, dysphonia, dystrophic, dystrophy).
5. Which of the following words does *not* pertain to vision? (myopia, oncologist, optician, optometrist)
6. Excessive thirst is (exogenous, hyperthermia, neoplasm, polydipsia).
7. Death of tissue is (diathermy, epilepsy, necrosis, pyoderma).
8. Absence of speech is (aphasia, aphonia, ectopic, hemiplegia).
9. Which of the following terms does *not* contain a prefix that indicates location? (mesonasal, postnasal, supratonsillar, tachycardia)
10. Sudden attacks of sleep occurring at intervals is called (bradyphasia, mycodermatitis, narcolepsy, photophobia).
11. Which of the following specialties deals particularly with problems of the elderly? (cryosurgery, gerontology, oncology, orthodontics)
12. A fever-producing agent is called a (pyoderma, pyogen, pyrogen, pyrophobia).
13. Which of the following terms does *not* contain a word part that indicates large or enlarged? (cardiomegaly, macrocephaly, microorganism, megalocyte)
14. The term electroencephalograph has something to do with recording the electrical impulses of the brain. Specifically, the term refers to the (instrument used, outcome, process itself, record produced).

F. Using word parts you have learned, write letters in the blanks to complete each term correctly.

1. Treatment of tissues by using cold temperatures is
   — — — —therapy.
2. A substance that can dissolve fibrous material is a
   fibro — — — — —.
3. A benign fatty tumor is a lip— — —.
4. Deficiency of oxygen results in a slightly bluish, slatelike color of the skin called — — — — —sis.
5. Treatment of disease by movement or exercise is
   — — — — — — —therapy.
6. A white blood cell is a — — — — —cyte.
7. Fear of death or of dead bodies is — — — — —phobia.
8. Inflammation of the skin is dermat — — — —.
9. Painful or difficult movement is — — —kinesia.
10. Any cell that ingests (eats) particulate matter is a
    — — — — —cyte.

11. Examination or viewing of small things is
micro __ __ __ __ __.
12. Under the skin is __ __ __ __dermic.

G. Write the medical term for which each meaning is given:

1. study of fungi _____

2. cancerous tumor _____

3. surgical crushing of a stone _____

4. abnormal preoccupation with fire _____

5. any disease of the eye _____

6. the study of cells _____

7. the origin or beginning of cancer _____

8. paralysis of all four extremities _____

Body Structure and Body Systems

4 Body Structure

OBJECTIVES

After completing Chapter 4, you will be able to

1. Write the meanings of the word parts presented in this chapter, choose their correct meanings when presented with several answers, and recognize and write the meanings of the word parts when they appear in medical terms.
2. Write the meanings and recognize the definitions of terms related to directional aspects of the body.
3. Choose the correct definitions for terms presented in this chapter that are related to body structures and write the appropriate terms when presented with their definitions.
4. Match terms related to body fluids with their descriptions and write the terms when presented with their definitions.
5. Choose the correct definitions for terms related to body cavities presented in this chapter and write the appropriate terms when presented with their definitions.

OUTLINE

THE ANATOMIC POSITION AND REFERENCE PLANES OF THE BODY
BODY CAVITIES
BODY STRUCTURES
BODY FLUIDS
COMPREHENSIVE REVIEW EXERCISES

THE ANATOMIC POSITION AND REFERENCE PLANES OF THE BODY

Anatomic[1] reference systems provide uniformity in regard to descriptions of the body. The **anatomic position** means that a person is standing erect with the arms at the side and the palms forward (Fig. 4–1). This position is used as a reference when describing the location or direction of various body structures or parts.

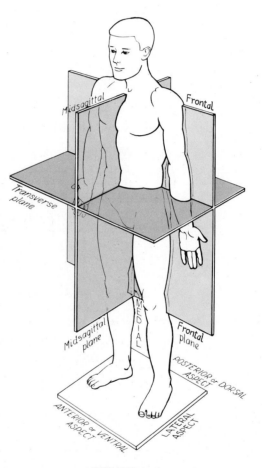

FIGURE 4–1

Anatomic position of body (*anterior view, palms forward*), with reference systems (planes and aspects). (Adapted from Jacob, S. W., Francone, C. A., and Lossow, W.J. : *Structure and Function in Man.* 5th ed. Philadelphia, W. B. Saunders, 1982.)

---

[1] an"ah tom'ik

Unless otherwise stated, all descriptions of location or position assume that the body is in the anatomic position. Commit to **memory** the following terms that relate to various directions of the body:

DIRECTIONAL TERMS

Term	Combining Form	Meaning
anterior[2]	anter/o	nearer to or toward the front; ventral
posterior[3]	poster/o	nearer to or toward the back; dorsal
ventral[4]	ventr/o	belly side; same as anterior surface in humans
dorsal[5]	dors/o	directed toward or situated on the back side; same as posterior surface in humans
medial,[6] median[7]	medi/o	middle or nearer the middle
lateral[8]	later/o	toward the side; denoting a position farther from the midline of the body or from a structure
superior[9]	super/o	uppermost or above
inferior[10]	infer/o	lowermost or below
proximal[11]	proxim/o	nearest the origin or point of attachment
distal[12]	dist/o	far or distant from the origin or point of attachment

[2] an tēr'e or
[3] pos tēr'e or
[4] ven'tral
[5] dor'sal
[6] me'de al
[7] me'de an

[8] lat'er al
[9] soo pēr'e or
[10] in fēr'e or
[11] prok'sĭ mal
[12] dis'tal

DIRECTIONAL TERMS
(Continued)

Term	Combining Form	Meaning
cephalad[13]	cephal/o	toward the head
caudad[14]	caud/o	toward the tail or in a posterior direction

PROGRAMMED LEARNING

Remember to cover the answers in the left column and to check them after you work each frame.

anterior	1. The body is facing forward in the anatomic position. Anterior means toward the front; therefore, the anatomic position is the _____ aspect or front of the body.
front	2. Antero/median[15] indicates the direction of _____ and toward the middle.
back	3. Posterior is the opposite of anterior. Posterior means directed toward or situated at the _____ .
back	4. Postero/medial[16] means situated in the middle of the _____ .
back	5. Postero/external[17] means situated toward the back and outer side. Postero/internal[18] means situated toward the _____ and the inner side.
front	6. In radiology, directional terms are used to specify the direction of the x-ray beam from its source to its exit surface before striking the film. In an antero/posterior[19] projection, the x-ray beam strikes the anterior aspect of the body first. In other words, the beam passes from the _____ of the body to the back.

[13] sef'ah lad
[14] kaw'dad
[15] an"ter o me'de an
[16] pos"ter o me'de an

[17] pos"ter o ek ster'nal
[18] pos"ter o in ter'nal
[19] an"ter o pos tēr'e or

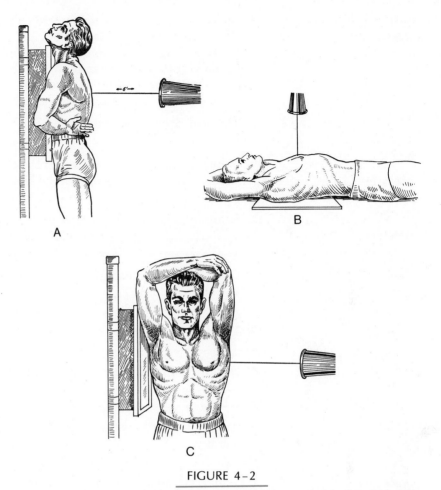

A

B

C

FIGURE 4-2

Directional terms pertaining to x-rays denote the direction of the beam from the x-ray source to its exit surface. *A,* Posteroanterior projection. The x-ray beam strikes the posterior aspect of the body first. *B,* Anteroposterior projection. The x-ray beam strikes the anterior aspect of the body first. *C,* Right lateral projection of the chest. Lateral x-ray projections are named according to the side of the patient nearer the x-ray film. (From Meschan, I.: *Radiographic Positioning and Related Anatomy.* 2nd ed. Philadelphia, W. B. Saunders, 1978.)

back

7. Postero/anterior[20] means from the posterior to the anterior surface—in other words, from _____ to front. (Figure 4-2 shows three radiographic positions.)

_____

_____

[20] pos"ter o an tēr'e or

back

8. Dorsal also means directed toward or situated on the back side. Dorso/ventral[21] pertains to the _____ and belly surfaces. Dorsoventral sometimes means passing from the back to the belly surface. For example, the path of a bullet resulting from a shot in the back could be described as dorsoventral.

ventral

9. The term for belly surface is _____.

anterior

10. In humans, the ventral surface is the same as the _____ aspect of the body.

posterior

11. Similarly, the dorsal surface in humans is the same as the _____ aspect of the body.

back

12. Dorso/lateral[22] means pertaining to the _____ and at the side.

side

13. That is because lateral means pertaining to the _____.

side

14. Postero/lateral[23] also means located behind and at the _____.

front

15. Antero/lateral[24] means situated in _____ and to one side.

side

16. Medio/lateral[25] means in the middle and to one _____.

medial
median

17. Two terms that mean middle are _____ and _____.

above

18. Superior means uppermost or situated above. Antero/superior[26] indicates in front and _____.

---

[21] dor″so ven′tral
[22] dor″so lat′er al
[23] pos″ter o lat′er al
[24] an″ter o lat′er al
[25] me″de o lat′er al
[26] an″ter o su pēr′e or

posterosuperior[27]	19. Using the combining form for posterior, build a word that means behind and above: _____
below	20. Inferior is the opposite of superior. In anatomy, inferior means situated _____.
middle	21. Infero/median[28] means situated in the _____ of the underside.
tail	22. Caudad means toward the tail. Caud/al[29] means pertaining to the _____, or to a tail-like structure. Sometimes it is also used to mean inferior in position.
near	23. Proximal describes the position of structures that are nearest their origin or point of attachment. The combining form proxim/o is used in words that refer to proximal, or _____.
nearer	24. The proximal end of the thigh bone joins with the hip bone. This means that the proximal end of the thigh bone is _____ the hip bone than the other end of the thigh bone.
far (distant) **distal**	25. Distal is the opposite of proximal. Distal means _____. It also means away from the origin or point of attachment. The lower end of the thigh bone is _____ to the hip bone.
distant	26. Distal is derived from the same word root as distant, and this should help you to remember the term. The combining form tel/e also means distant. A tele/cardiogram,[30] for instance, is a tracing of the electrical impulses of the heart recorded by a machine _____ from the patient.
	27. With a telecardiogram, the cardiologist and the patient may be in different cities. Telecardiograms can be sent by telephone.

---

[27] pos"te ro soo pēr'e or
[28] in"fer o me'de an
[29] kaw'dal
[30] tel ĕ kar'de o gram

EXERCISE I

Review some of the terms that have been used to indicate direction. Write a word in each blank to complete the table correctly. (The first one has been done as an example.)

Combining Form	Anatomic Term	Basic Meaning
1. anter/o	anterior	front
2. caud/o	_____	_____
3. dist/o	_____	_____
4. dors/o	_____	_____
5. infer/o	_____	_____
6. later/o	_____	_____
7. medi/o	_____	_____
	or _____	
8. poster/o	_____	_____
9. proxim/o	_____	_____
10. super/o	_____	_____
11. ventr/o	_____	_____

(Check your answers with the solutions in the back of the book.)

BODY CAVITIES

The body has two major cavities, which are spaces within the body that contain internal organs. The two principal body cavities are the **dorsal cavity,** located near the posterior aspect of the body, and the **ventral cavity,** located near the anterior aspect. Both cavities are subdivided as shown in Figure 4–3. The dorsal cavity is divided into the **cranial**[31] and **spinal**[32] **cavities.** The cranial cavity contains the brain and the spinal cavity contains the spinal cord and the beginnings of the spinal nerves. The other principal body cavity is the ventral cavity. Large organs contained in the ventral cavity are called **viscera.**[33] The ventral cavity is subdivided into the **thoracic**[34] (chest) cavity and the **abdominopelvic**[35] (abdominal and pelvic) cavity. The muscular **diaphragm**[36] divides the thoracic and abdominopelvic cavities.

---

[31] kra′ne al
[32] spi′nal
[33] vis′er ah

[34] tho ras′ik
[35] ab dom″ĭ no pel′vik
[36] di′ah fram

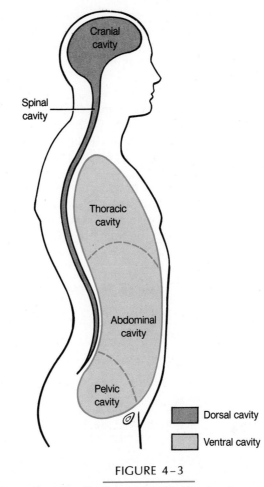

FIGURE 4–3

The body has two principal body cavities, the dorsal and ventral cavities. Each is subdivided further. (From Leonard, P. C.: *Building a Medical Vocabulary*. 2nd ed. Philadelphia, W. B. Saunders, 1988.)

The abdominopelvic cavity can be thought of as a single cavity or as two cavities, the abdominal and pelvic cavities, although no wall separates them. A membrane called the **peritoneum**[37] lines the abdominopelvic cavity and invests the internal organs. Peritoneum, like all serous membranes, secretes a lubricating fluid that allows the organs to glide against one another or against the cavity wall. A stick-

[37] per″ĭ to ne′um

ing together of two structures that are normally separated is called an **adhesion.**[38] Abdominal[39] adhesions are usually caused by inflammation or trauma (injury), and are treated surgically if they cause intestinal obstruction or excessive discomfort.

BODY STRUCTURES

The **cell** is the smallest functional unit of the human body and, in fact, of all organisms. Cells comprise the tissues of the body, which in turn make up organs. Each body system is a group of organs that work together for a specific purpose. The human organism has many body systems (Fig. 4–4).

Many body structures will be discussed elsewhere in this book. The following list includes several terms that either do not pertain to a particular body system or may pertain to more than one system. Commit the following list to **memory.**

SELECTED COMBINING FORMS THAT RELATE TO BODY STRUCTURES

Combining Form	Meaning
abdomin/o	abdomen
acr/o	extremities (arms and legs)
blephar/o	eyelid
cephal/o	head
chir/o	hand
cyst/o	cyst, bladder, or sac
dactyl/o	digit (toes, fingers, or both)
lapar/o	abdominal wall
omphal/o	umbilicus[40] (navel)
onych/o	nail
pelv/i	pelvis
periton/o	peritoneum
som/a, somat/o	body
thorac/o	chest

[38] ad he'zhun
[39] ab dom'ĭ nal

[40] um bil'ĭ kus, um"bĭ li'kus

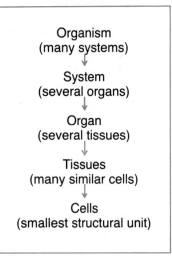

FIGURE 4-4

Structural relationships within the body. There are many types of cells, such as nerve cells, blood cells, and epithelial cells. Examples of tissues are connective, skeletal, muscular, and nervous tissues. The liver, kidney, lung, stomach, and heart are types of organs. Body systems include the circulatory, skeletal, digestive, urinary, and respiratory systems. (Adapted from Miller, M. J.: *Pathophysiology*. Philadelphia, W. B. Saunders, 1983.)

The abdomen[41] is the portion of the body trunk that is located between the chest and the pelvis. **Abdomino/centesis**[42] (abdomin/o, abdomen, + centesis, surgical puncture), usually called **abdominal paracentesis**,[43] is a surgical procedure that is performed to remove excess fluids (ascites[44]) from the abdominal cavity or to inject a therapeutic agent. **Peritonitis**[45] (periton/o, peritoneum, + -itis, inflammation) can result if infectious microorganisms gain access by way of operative incisions or by the rupture or perforation of viscera or associated structures (as in rupture of the appendix). Microorganisms can also spread to the peritoneum from the blood stream or lymphatic vessels.

Incision of the abdominal wall is called **laparo/tomy**[46] (lapar/o, abdominal wall, + -tomy, incision). Laparotomy is another way of

---

[41] ab do'men, ab'do men   [44] ah si'tēz
[42] ab dom"ĭ no sen te'sis   [45] per"ĭ to ni'tis
[43] par"ah sen te'sis   [46] lap ah rot'o me

saying an abdominal operation. Several surgical procedures involve incision of the abdominal wall, some of which are described:

laparocholecystotomy[47] (lapar/o, abdominal wall, + cholecyst/o, gallbladder, + -tomy, incision): incision into the gallbladder through the abdominal wall

laparocolostomy[48] (lapar/o + col/o, large intestine, + -stomy, new opening): formation of a permanent opening into the colon (large intestine) through the abdominal wall

laparocystotomy[49] (lapar/o + cyst/o, cyst, + -tomy): abdominal incision to remove a cyst or an embryo that has implanted outside the uterus (synonym: laparocystectomy[50])

laparogastrotomy[51] (lapar/o + gastr/o, stomach, + -tomy): abdominal incision into the stomach

laparohepatotomy[52] (lapar/o + hepat/o, liver, + -tomy): incision of the liver through the abdominal wall

laparohysterectomy[53] (lapar/o + hyster/o, uterus, + -ectomy, excision): removal of the uterus through an incision in the abdominal wall

laparohysteropexy[54] (lapar/o + hyster/o + -pexy, surgical fixation): attachment of the uterus to the abdominal wall

laparorrhaphy[55] (lapar/o + -rrhaphy, suture): suture of the abdominal wall

laparoscopy[56] (lapar/o + -scopy, visual examination): abdominal exploration employing a laparoscope,[57] an instrument used to view the interior of the abdomen (laparoscopy is a type of **endoscopy**,[58] inspection of body organs or cavities using an endoscope,[59] a device that uses fiberoptic techniques to permit visual imaging around corners)

laparosplenotomy[60] (lapar/o + splen/o, spleen, + -tomy): incision of the spleen through an abdominal operation

NEW COMBINING FORMS USED

Combining Form	Meaning
cholecyst/o	gallbladder
col/o	colon (large intestine)
gastr/o	stomach
hepat/o	liver
hyster/o	uterus
splen/o	spleen

---

[47] lap"ah ro ko"le sis tot'o me
[48] lap"ah ro ko los'to me
[49] lap"ah ro sis tot'o me
[50] lap"ah ro sis tek'to me
[51] lap"ah ro gas trot'o me
[52] lap"ah ro hep"ah tot'o me
[53] lap"ah ro his"ter ek'to me

[54] lap"ah ro his"ter o pek'se
[55] lap ah ror'ah fe
[56] lap"ah ros'ko pe
[57] lap'ah ro skōp"
[58] en dos'ko pe
[59] en'do skōp
[60] lap"ah ro sple not'o me

The pelvis is the lower portion of the body trunk. The word pelvis can refer to any basinlike structure, so you will also see it in other terms (e.g., the renal pelvis, a funnel-shaped structure within the kidney). **Pelvimetry**[61] (pelv/i, pelvis, + -metry, measurement) is the measurement of the dimensions and capacity of the pelvis. It is seldom done anymore, because the procedure usually involves the use of x-rays. The instrument used in pelvimetry is a **pelvimeter.**[62] A **cephalopelvic**[63] **disproportion** is a situation in which the head of the fetus is too large for the pelvis of the mother. In such cases vaginal delivery is difficult or impossible. Cephalopelvic (cephal/o, head, + pelv/i, pelvis) is a term that pertains to the head of the fetus and the maternal pelvis.

Omphalos is Greek for the umbilicus, or navel. Many new terms can be formed using omphal/o with various suffixes that you have already learned. **Omphalic**[64] means concerning the umbilicus. **Umbilical**[65] also means pertaining to the umbilicus. An inflamed condition of the navel is **omphal/itis.**[66] Congenital hernia of the navel is **omphalo/cele.**[67] Rupture of the navel is **omphalo/rrhexis,**[68] and umbilical hemorrhage is **omphalo/rrhagia.**[69]

Thoracic means pertaining to the chest, because thorac/o means thorax[70] or chest. Thoracic surgery is another way of saying chest surgery. Surgical puncture of the chest wall for aspiration of fluids could be called thoracocentesis,[71] but **thoracentesis**[72] is the more commonly used term.

EXERCISE II

Using what you have just learned, and word parts studied in previous chapters, circle the correct answer to complete each sentence.

1. The combining form that means arms and legs is (acr/o, chir/o, cyst/o, omphal/o).
2. The combining form blephar/o means (extremities, eyelid, brain, head).
3. The combining form that means abdomen is (pelv/i, pelv/o, abdomen/o, abdomin/o).

---

[61] pel vim′ĕ tre
[62] pel vim′ĕ ter
[63] sef″ah lo pel′vik
[64] om fal′ik
[65] um bil′ĭ kal
[66] om″fah li′tis

[67] om″fah lo sēl′
[68] om″fah lo rek′sis
[69] om″fah lo ra′je ah
[70] tho′raks
[71] tho″rah ko sen te′sis
[72] tho″rah sen te′sis

4. The combining form onych/o means (head, bladder, digit, nail).
5. The combining form for a membrane that lines the abdominopelvic cavity is (omphal/o, lapar/o, somat/o, periton/o).
6. The combining form somat/o means (sleep, body, toes or fingers, cyst).
7. The combining form omphal/o means (umbilicus, abdominal wall, head, chest).
8. The combining form col/o means (gallbladder, cyst, large intestine, liver).
9. The combining form hyster/o means (uterus, abdominal wall, spleen, pelvis).
10. The combining form for the stomach is (cholecyst/o, hepat/o, gastr/o, splen/o).
11. Pain in the thorax, distinguished from chest pain caused by angina pectoris, a heart condition, is (thoracocentesis, thoracoschisis, thoracodynia, thoracectomy).
12. Surgical incision of the chest wall is (thoracotomy, thoracostomy, thoracostenosis, thoracolysis).
13. Diagnostic examination of the chest cavity is (pleurotomy, pleurectomy, thoracometry, thoracoscopy).
14. Plastic surgery of the chest in which portions of the ribs are removed to cause diseased areas of the lung to collapse is (thoracolysis, thoracoplasty, thoracalgia, thoracopathy).

(Check your answers.)

Several words contain the word part cephal/o, meaning head. **Cephalometry**[73] (cephal/o + -metry) is measurement of the dimensions of the head. **Cephalalgia**[74] and **cephalodynia**[75] (cephal/o + -algia or -dynia, pain) mean pain in the head or headache. Cephalad refers to the head or toward the head.

You learned previously that ophthalm/o means eye. Blephar/o refers to the eyelid. Your knowledge of suffixes should enable you to recognize and write many new terms using blephar/o in the following exercise.

EXERCISE III   *Using words or word parts you have learned, write letters in the blanks to complete each sentence correctly.*

1. Blephar/al[76] means pertaining to the __ __ __ __ __ __.

---

[73] sef"ah lom'ĕ tre   [75] sef"ah lo din'e ah
[74] sef"ah lal'je ah   [76] blef'ah ral

2. Blephar/itis[77] is __ __ __ __ __ __ __ __ __ __ __ __ __ __ of the eyelid. Blepharitis could lead to __ __ __ __ __ __ __ ede-ma, swelling of the eyelids. There are other causes of blephar-edema,[78] such as crying.
3. Blepharoplegia[79] is __ __ __ __ __ __ __ __ __ of an eyelid.
4. Blepharoptosis[80] is prolapse or __ __ __ __ __ __ __ of the upper eyelid.
5. Twitching of the eyelid is blepharo __ __ __ __ __.
6. Plastic surgery performed on the eyelid is __ __ __ __ __ __ __ __ __ __ __ __ __.
7. Surgical incision of the eyelid is __ __ __ __ __ __ __ __ __ __ __ __.

(Check your answers.)

Extremities of the body are the arms and legs. The combining form acr/o is used to refer to the extremities. In working the following exercise, you will learn new terms that pertain to the arms and legs.

EXERCISE IV

Write letters in the blanks to complete each sentence correctly.

1. Acro/cyanosis[81] is cyanosis of the extremities. In acrocyanosis, the arms and legs seem to be the color __ __ __ __.
2. Acrodermatitis[82] is dermatitis of the extremities. In other words, the __ __ __ __ of the arms and legs is inflamed.
3. Acr/al[83] pertains to the __ __ __ __ __ __ __ __ __ __ __ __ __.
4. Acrohypothermy[84] is abnormal coldness of the extremities. Translated literally, acro/hypo/thermy means below normal __ __ __ __ in the extremities.
5. Acro/megaly[85] is a disorder in which there is abnormal enlargement of the __ __ __ __ __ __ __ __ __ __ __ of the body, including the nose, jaws, fingers, and toes, caused by hypersecretion of growth hormone after maturity.

(Check your answers.)

---

[77] blef"ah ri'tis
[78] blef"ar e de'mah
[79] blef"ah ro ple'je ah
[80] blef"ah ro to'sis
[81] ak"ro si ah no'sis
[82] ak"ro der"mah ti'tis
[83] ak'ral
[84] ak"ro hi"po ther'me
[85] ak"ro meg'ah le

A finger or toe is a digit. The combining form dactyl/o is often used in words that pertain to the fingers and toes. **Dactylography**[86] is the study of fingerprints. **Dactylospasm**[87] means cramping of a finger or toe. Inflammation of the bones of the fingers and toes is **dactylitis.**[88]

Chiro/pody[89] means pertaining to the hands and feet. It is also the art or profession of a chiropodist,[90] one who treats corns, bunions, and other afflictions of the hands and feet. Cramping of the hand, such as writer's cramp, is **chiro/spasm.**[91] Plastic surgery of the hand is **chiro/plasty.**[92]

The combining form onych/o refers to the nails. An **onychophagist**[93] (onych/o, nails, + phag/o, eat, + -ist, one who) habitually bites the nails. The following exercise will help you to learn new terms that use the combining form onych/o.

EXERCISE V

Write the correct answer in each blank space.

1. Onycho/malacia[94] is _____ of the nails.
2. An onych/oma[95] is a _____ of the nail or nail bed.
3. Onycho/myc/osis[96] is a disease of the _____ caused by a _____.
4. Any disease of the nails is called an _____.
5. Surgical removal of the nail is _____. (This term also means declawing of an animal.)

(Check your answers.)

BODY FLUIDS

Several word parts that relate to body fluids are presented below. After you complete the programmed study that follows this list, you should be able to recognize the meanings of the word parts.

---

[86] dak″tĭ log′rah fe
[87] dak′tĭ lo spazm
[88] dak″tĭ li′tis
[89] ki rop′o de
[90] ki rop′o dist
[91] ki′ro spazm

[92] ki′ro plas″te
[93] on″ĭ kof′ah jist
[94] on″ĭ ko mah la′she ah
[95] on″ĭ ko′mah
[96] on″ĭ ko mi ko′sis

SELECTED WORD PARTS THAT PERTAIN TO BODY FLUIDS

Combining Form or Word Part	Meaning
crin/o, -crine	secrete
dacry/o, lacrim/o	tear, tearing, crying
-emia, hem/a, hem/o, hemat/o	blood
hidr/o	sweat or perspiration
hydr/o	water
lymph/o	lymph (sometimes refers to the lymphatics)
muc/o	mucus
py/o	pus
sial/o	saliva (sometimes refers to salivary glands)
ur/o	urine (sometimes refers to the urinary tract)

PROGRAMMED LEARNING

Remember to check your answers after working each frame.

crying or tearing	1. The combining forms dacry/o and lacrim/o mean tear, as in crying. The lacrimal[97] gland produces fluid that keeps the eye moist. Tears are lacrimal fluid. If more lacrimal fluid is produced than can be removed, we say that the person is _____ .
tears	2. Lacrimation[98] refers to crying, or the discharge of _____ .
inflammation	3. Ophthalmitis[99] may lead to excessive lacrimation. Ophthalm/itis is _____ of the eye.

[97] lak′rĭ mal
[98] lak″rĭ ma′shun
[99] of″thal mi′tis

stone or calculus	4. Calculi (concretions) sometimes form in the lacrimal passages. A dacryo/lith[100] is a lacrimal _____. Dacryoliths are also called tear stones.
lacrimal stones	5. Dacryo/lith/iasis[101] is the presence of _____ _____.
dacryocyst	6. The dacryo/cyst[102] is the tear sac. The dacryocyst collects lacrimal fluid. Another name for the tear sac is _____.
inflammation	7. Dacryo/cyst/itis[103] is _____ of the tear sac.
dacryolith	8. Write the word that means tear stone: _____
sialolith	9. Stones can also occur in a salivary gland or duct. The combining form sial/o is used to form words that pertain to a salivary gland or to the fluid of these glands, called saliva.[104] Use dacryo/lith[105] as a model to write a word that means a salivary calculus: _____
salivary	10. Sialo/graphy[106] is x-ray of the ducts of the _____ glands. Sialography sometimes demonstrates the presence of calculi in the salivary ducts.
inside	11. In addition to salivary glands, the body contains many other types of glands. On the basis of the presence or absence of ducts, glands are classified as exocrine[107] or endocrine[108] glands. You previously learned that endo- means _____. The prefix exo- in this case means outside.
	12. The combining form crin/o and the suffix -crine mean secrete. Exo/crine glands have ducts that carry their secretions to an epithelial surface, sometimes to the outside (e.g., sweat glands

---

[100] dak're o lith"
[101] dak"re o lith i'ah sis
[102] dak're o sist"
[103] dak"re o sis ti'tis
[104] sah li'vah

[105] dak're o lith"
[106] si"ah log'rah fe
[107] ek'so krin
[108] en'do krīn, en'do krin

exocrine

secrete perspiration onto the skin surface). Salivary glands also have ducts. Are salivary glands exocrine or endocrine glands? _____

---

endocrine

13. Endocrine glands are ductless and secrete their hormones into the bloodstream. There are many ductless glands, including the sex glands, the thyroid,[109] and the adrenal[110] glands. Ductless glands are classified as _____ glands.

---

sweat

14. Sweat glands are also called sudoriferous[111] glands, because the Latin word *sudor* means sweat. The combining form for sweat that you will use, however, is hidr/o. Hidr/osis[112] means the formation and excretion of _____. A second meaning of hidrosis is excessive sweating, but diaphoresis[113] is the term that is usually used to mean excessive sweating.

---

sweat gland

15. Remembering that aden/o means gland, hidr/aden/itis[114] is inflammation of a _____ _____. (Notice that when hidr/o is joined with aden/o, the o is dropped from hidr/o to make it easier to pronounce.)

---

hidradenoma[115]

16. Now write a word that means tumor of a sweat gland: _____

---

water

17. The combining form hydr/o means water. Do not confuse hydr/o and hidr/o. Remembering that a water *hydrant* is spelled with a *y* might help. Hydro/therapy[116] refers to treatment using _____.

---

18. Hydrophobia[117] is another name for rabies, a viral disease transmitted by the bite of an infected animal. The disease was given the name hydrophobia after it was observed that rabid animals avoid water. It was later learned that they avoid water because the muscles of the throat are paralyzed and they

---

[109] thi′roid
[110] ah dre′nal
[111] su″do rif′er us
[112] hi dro′sis
[113] di″ah fo re′sis

[114] hi″drad ĕ ni′tis
[115] hi″drad ĕ no′mah
[116] hi″dro ther′ah pe
[117] hi″dro fo′be ah

fear, water	cannot swallow. Translated literally, hydrophobia means an abnormal _____ of _____.
hidr/o	19. The combining form for sweat or perspiration is _____.
blood	20. There are several word parts that mean blood. Hematology[118] is the study of blood, blood-forming tissues, and their physiology and pathology. Translated literally, hemato/logy is the study of _____
blood tumor	21. A hemat/oma[119] is a localized collection of blood, usually clotted, in an organ, space, or tissue, that results from a rupture in the wall of a blood vessel. The word *hematoma* is derived from the old meaning of tumor, a swelling, because there is a raised area wherever a hematoma occurs. Translated literally, hemat/oma means _____ _____.
blood	22. Hemo/dialysis[120] is the process of diffusing _____ through a semipermeable membrane to remove toxic materials from the body of those with impaired kidney function.
blood, destruction	23. If you break hemo/lysis into its component parts, hem/o means _____ and -lysis means _____. Hemolysis is actually the destruction of red blood cells with the liberation of their red pigment, hemoglobin.
blood	24. Globins[121] are types of proteins; therefore, hemo/globin[122] is a type of protein found in _____. (In humans, the hemoglobin is located in the red blood cells.) Hemoglobin carries oxygen to cells throughout the body and exchanges oxygen for waste carbon dioxide.
	25. Anemia[123] is a condition in which the blood is deficient in red

[118] hem″ah tol′o je
[119] hem″ah to′mah
[120] he″mo di al′ĭ sis
[121] glo′binz
[122] he′mo glo″bin
[123] ah ne′me ah

no, or without	blood cells, hemoglobin, or both. Translated literally, an/emia means _____ blood.
-emia	26. No one can live without blood, however, so some modification of the actual meaning of the word parts in anemia is necessary. The suffix in anemia that means blood is _____ .
blood	27. Leuk/emia[124] was so named because of the large number of white cells in the _____ of patients with the disease. Leukemia is a malignant disease of the blood-forming organs.
deficiency	28. You learned in an earlier chapter that -penia means deficiency. Leuko/penia is a _____ of white blood cells.
blood	29. Hemat/uria[125] is _____ in the urine.
urine	30. The combining form ur/o means urine. Translated literally, an/uria[126] means without _____. Production of less than 100 ml of urine in 24 hours constitutes anuria.
polyuria[127]	31. Using poly- and uria, write a word that means excessive urination: _____
lymph	32. Lymph[128] is another type of body fluid. It is a transparent fluid found in lymphatic vessels. The lymphatic[129] system (also called the lymphatics) collects tissue fluid from all parts of the body and returns the fluids to the blood circulation. Lymph/o usually refers to the lymphatics but sometimes refers to its fluid, _____ .
mucus	33. The combining form muc/o means mucus. Mucoid[130] means resembling _____ .

[124] loo ke′me ah
[125] hem″ah tu′re ah
[126] ah nu′re ah
[127] pol″e u′re ah

[128] limf
[129] lim fat′ik
[130] mu′koid

mucous

34. Mucous[131] also means resembling mucus. Notice the slight difference in the spelling of mucous and mucus. Mucous also means secreting mucus or depending on the presence of mucus. Two adjectives that mean resembling mucus are mucoid and _____ .

mucous

35. Membranes that line passages and cavities that communicate with the air are called mucous membranes. A mucous membrane is also called a mucosa.[132] Mucous membranes usually contain mucus-secreting cells. Passages and cavities that communicate with the air are lined with _____ membranes.

mucus

36. Muco/lytic[133] agents break up or destroy _____ , as in the case of certain diseases (e.g., bronchial asthma[134]).

pus

37. Pus is a type of body fluid that is the liquid product of inflammation. The combining form py/o means pus. Py/uria[135] is _____ in the urine.

pus

38. Pyo/genic[136] microorganisms are those that produce _____ .

EXERCISE VI

Match the word parts in the left column with their meanings in the right column (the choices on the right may be used more than once).

_____ 1. crin/o	A. urine
_____ 2. dacry/o	B. lymph
_____ 3. -emia	C. tear
_____ 4. hemat/o	D. blood
_____ 5. hidr/o	E. perspiration
_____ 6. hydr/o	F. water
_____ 7. lacrim/o	G. mucus
_____ 8. lymph/o	H. pus
_____ 9. muc/o	I. saliva
_____ 10. py/o	J. secrete
_____ 11. sial/o	
_____ 12. ur/o	

---

[131] mu′kus
[132] mu ko′sah
[133] mu″ko lit′ik

[134] brong′ke al az′mah
[135] pi u′re ah
[136] pi″o jen′ik

Comprehensive Review Exercises

WORK THE FOLLOWING EXERCISES TO TEST YOUR UNDERSTANDING OF THE
MATERIAL IN CHAPTER 4. IT IS BEST TO WORK ALL THE REVIEW EXERCISES
BEFORE CHECKING YOUR ANSWERS.

A. Use one of the following words to correctly complete the sentences.

abdominopelvic   peritoneum   ventral
cranial   spinal   viscera
dorsal   thoracic

The two principal body cavities are the (1) _____

cavity, located near the posterior aspect of the body, and the

(2) _____ cavity, located near the anterior aspect.

Each of these cavities is subdivided into smaller ones. The

(3) _____ cavity contains the spinal cord and the

beginnings of the spinal nerves. The (4) _____ cavity

contains the brain. The ventral cavity is subdivided into the

(5) _____ or chest cavity and the (6) _____

cavity. Large organs contained in the ventral cavity are called

(7) _____. A serous membrane called the

(8) _____ lines the abdominopelvic cavity and in-

vests the internal organs.

**B. Match the terms in the left column with the directional terms in
the right column.**

_____ 1. caudal   A. above
_____ 2. cephalad   B. back
_____ 3. distal   C. far
_____ 4. dorsal   D. front
_____ 5. proximal   E. head
                         F. near
                         G. tail

C. Write the correct answer in each blank space.

1. Anteromedian indicates the position of _____ and
   toward the middle.

2. Posteromedial means situated in the middle of the

   _____ .

3. In an anteroposterior projection, the x-ray beam strikes the
   _____ aspect of the body first.

4. Dorsoventral pertains to the back and _____ surfaces.

5. Posterolateral means located behind and to the _____ .

6. Mediolateral means in the _____ and to one

   _____ .

7. Anterosuperior indicates in front and _____ .

8. Inferomedian means situated in the _____ of the

   _____ .

**D. Write the meaning of each underlined word part in the blank
spaces.**

   1. hemoglobin _____

   2. leukemia _____ ; _____

   3. polyuria _____ ; _____ ;

      _____

   4. acral _____ ; _____

   5. hydrotherapy _____

   6. hematopoiesis _____

   7. onychoma _____ ; _____

   8. laparocholecystotomy _____ ; _____

   9. telecardiogram _____ ; _____ ;

      _____

   10. omphalic _____ ; _____

E. Circle the correct answer to complete each sentence.

   1. A deficiency of white blood cells is (erythrocytosis, hemolysis,
      leukopenia, cyanosis).

   2. A sticking together of two structures that are normally separated
      is called an (ascites, abdominal paracentesis, adhesion, anuria).

   3. Abdominal exploration that uses a special instrument to view the
      interior of the abdomen is (laparocolostomy, laparohysteropexy,
      laparorrhaphy, laparoscopy).

4. Measurement of the dimensions and capacity of the pelvis is (cephalopelvic disproportion, pelvimeter, pelvimetry, umbilical).

5. Surgical puncture of the chest wall for aspiration of fluids is (thoracic, thoracentesis, thoracodynia, thoracoplasty).

6. Congenital hernia of the navel is (omphalitis, omphalorrhexis, omphalorrhagia, omphalocele).

7. A headache is (cephalodynia, hematoma, lacrimation, peritonitis).

8. Sagging of the eyelid is (blepharal, blepharedema, blepharitis, blepharoptosis).

9. Inflammation of the skin of the arms and legs is (acrocyanosis, acrodermatitis, acrohypothermy, acromegaly).

10. Cramping of a finger or toe is (chiropody, chirospasm, dactylitis, dactylospasm).

F. Write letters in the blanks to complete each sentence correctly.

1. Surgical removal of the nail is __ __ __ __ __ectomy.

2. The presence of lacrimal stones is __ __ __ __ __ __lithiasis.

3. Inflammation of a sweat gland is __ __ __ __adenitis.

4. Ductless glands that secrete hormones into the bloodstream are __ __ __ __ __ __ __ __ __ glands.

5. __ __ __ __ __graphy is x-ray of the ducts of the salivary glands.

6. __ __ __ __ __ __ __ __ __ __ is another name for a tear sac.

7. A condition in which the blood is deficient in erythrocytes, hemoglobin, or both is __ __ __ __ __ __.

8. The destruction of erythrocytes with the liberation of hemoglobin is __ __ __ __ __ __ __ __ __.

9. Pus in the urine is __ __uria.

10. __ __ __ __ __ __ __ __ __ agents are those that break up or destroy mucus.

G. Write the medical term for which each meaning is given:

1. incision of the chest wall _____

2. measurement of the head _____

3. inflammation of the eyelid _____

4. surgical repair of the hand _____

5. inflammation of the bones of the fingers or toes _____

6. morbid softening of the nails _____

The Skeletal and Muscular Systems

OBJECTIVES

After completing Chapter 5, you will be able to

1. Write the meaning of the word parts pertaining to the skeletal and muscular systems given in this chapter and choose their correct meanings when presented with several answers.
2. Write the scientific and common names of major bones of the body.
3. Name and describe the general locations of the five different types of vertebrae.
4. Analyze terms related to the skeletal and muscular systems, select the appropriate response when presented with several answers, and write the terms when presented with their definitions.
5. Match the diseases or disorders presented in this chapter with their descriptions.

OUTLINE

FUNCTIONS OF THE SKELETAL AND MUSCULAR SYSTEMS
MAJOR BONES OF THE BODY
THE SPINE
    Injury to the Spine
    Malformations of the Spine
    Other Spinal Disorders
    Other Terms Related to the Spine
CARTILAGE
ARTICULATIONS AND ASSOCIATED STRUCTURES
MUSCLES AND ASSOCIATED STRUCTURES
DISEASES, DISORDERS, AND DIAGNOSTIC TERMS
COMPREHENSIVE REVIEW EXERCISES

FUNCTIONS OF THE SKELETAL AND MUSCULAR SYSTEMS

The skeletal and muscular systems cooperate to provide protection, support, and movement for the body. **Orthopedics**[1] is that branch of medicine involved in the prevention and correction of deformities or diseases of the muscular and skeletal systems, especially those of the bones, muscles, joints, ligaments, and tendons. Ortho/ped/ics (orth/o, straight, + ped/o, child, + -ic, pertaining to) was so named because the **orthopedist**[2] originally aligned children's bones and corrected deformities. Today, however, an orthopedist specializes in disorders of the bones and associated structures in people of all ages.

The **skeleton,** composed of bone and cartilage, **is the framework of the body,** and provides a place for the attachment of tendons, ligaments, and muscles. In addition, bones serve as storage for mineral salts and are important in **hematopoiesis**[3] (hemat/o, blood, + -poiesis, production). **Muscles effect movement** of an organ or part of the body by contracting and relaxing. Because of the close association of the body's skeleton and muscles, the two systems are often referred to as one, as in **musculoskeletal**[4] (muscul/o, muscle) disorders. Muscles are also closely related to the nervous system, because nerve impulses stimulate the muscles to contract.

FIGURE 5–1

Bones of the skeletal system. The cranium (1) protects the brain and forms the framework of the face. The clavicle (2) is attached to the upper end of the sternum (3). Also attached to the sternum are the ribs (4), which support the chest wall and protect the lungs and heart. The vertebrae (5) protect the spinal cord. The scapula (6) is a large triangular bone that joins the upper end of the longest bone of the arm, the humerus (7), by muscles and tendons. The bones of the forearm are the ulna (8) and the radius (9). The wrist is composed of eight carpal bones, or carpals (10). The bones of the palm are the metacarpals (11) and the bones of the fingers are the phalanges (12). The major bones of the pelvis are the ilium (13) and the ischium (14). The longest bone of the leg is the femur (15). The kneecap, called the patella (16), overlaps the bottom end of the femur and protects the knee joint, where the femur and tibia (17) meet. The other bone of the lower leg is the fibula (18). The ankle is composed of seven tarsal bones, or tarsals (19). The bones of the feet are the metatarsals (20). Like the bones of the fingers, those of the toes are called phalanges (21). (Modified from Liebgott, B.: *The Anatomical Basis of Dentistry.* Philadelphia, W. B. Saunders, 1982.)

---

[1] or"tho pe'diks
[2] or"tho pe'dist
[3] hem"ah to poi e'sis
[4] mus"ku lo skel'ĕ tal

MAJOR BONES OF THE BODY

The adult human skeleton has 206 named bones; the major bones are shown in Figure 5–1. Write the names of the bones on the figure as you read the accompanying paragraphs.

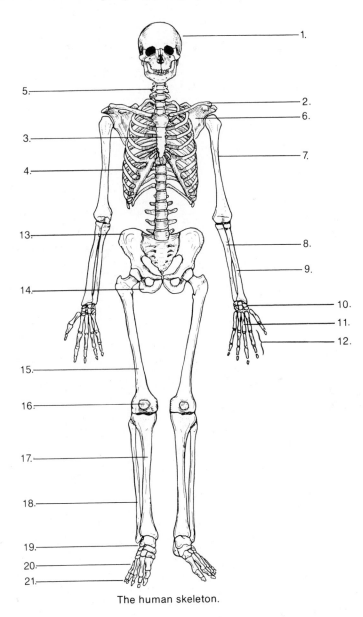

FIGURE 5–1

See legend on opposite page

The human skeleton.

The following is a list of the combining forms for the major bones of the body, as well as their common names (when appropriate). Commit this information to **memory.**

**MAJOR BONES OF
THE BODY**

Bone	Combining Form	Common Name
cranium[5]	crani/o	skull
bones of the chest:		
clavicle[6]	clavicul/o	collarbone
costa[7]	cost/o	rib
scapula[8]	scapul/o	shoulder blade
sternum[9]	stern/o	breastbone
vertebra[10] (pl., vertebrae)	vertebr/o or spondyl/o	bone(s) of the spinal column
bones of the pelvis:		
ilium[11]	ili/o	
ischium[12]	ischi/o	hip bones
pubis[13]	pub/o	
bones of the arm and hand:		
humerus[14]	humer/o	
radius[15]	radi/o	
ulna[16]	uln/o	
carpals[17]	carp/o	wrist bones
metacarpals[18]	metacarp/o	
phalanges[19]	phalang/o	bones of the fingers
bones of the legs and feet:		
femur[20]	femor/o	thigh bone
patella[21]	patell/o	kneecap
fibula[22]	fibul/o	
tibia[23]	tibi/o	
tarsals[24]	tars/o*	ankle bones
metatarsals[25]	metatars/o	
phalanges	phalang/o	bones of the toes

* Tars/o refers to the ankle (the tarsus) or to the ankle bones. Tars/o also means the edge of the eyelid, because a second meaning of tarsus is "a curved plate of dense white fibrous tissue forming the supporting structure of the eyelid."

[5] kra'ne um
[6] klav'ĭ kal
[7] kos'tah
[8] skap'u lah
[9] ster'num
[10] ver'tĕ brah
[11] il'e um
[12] is'ke um
[13] pu'bis
[14] hu'mer us
[15] ra'de us
[16] ul'nah
[17] kar'palz
[18] met"ah kar'palz
[19] fah lan' jēz
[20] fe'mur
[21] pah tel'ah
[22] fib'u lah
[23] tib'e ah
[24] tahr'salz
[25] met"ah tar'salz

EXERCISE I

Match the names of bones in the left column with their common names in the right column. (The choices on the right may be used more than once).

_____ 1. carpals	A. ankle bones
_____ 2. clavicle	B. bones of the fingers or toes
_____ 3. cranium	C. breastbone
_____ 4. femur	D. collarbone
_____ 5. ilium	E. hip bone
_____ 6. ischium	F. kneecap
_____ 7. patella	G. shoulder blade
_____ 8. phalanges	H. skull
_____ 9. pubis	I. thigh bone
_____ 10. scapula	J. wrist bones
_____ 11. sternum	
_____ 12. tarsals	

(Check your answers with the solutions in the back of the book.)

EXERCISE II

Write the combining form that corresponds to each bone.

1. femur _____
2. fibula _____
3. humerus _____
4. radius _____
5. rib _____
6. tibia _____
7. ulna _____
8. vertebra _____ or _____
9. Of the eight bones that are listed above, which are bones of the arm?

   _____

10. Of the eight bones that are listed above, which are bones of the leg?

    _____

PROGRAMMED LEARNING

*Remember to cover the answers in the left column and to check them
after you work each frame.*

---

skull

1. The common name for cranium is _____. A second meaning of cranium is the specific portion of the skull that encloses and protects the brain. The skull is composed of cranial bones, facial bones, and teeth.

---

crani/o

2. Cranium usually refers to the skull. The combining form for cranium is _____.

---

skull (cranium)

3. Cranio/cele[26] is a hernial protrusion of the brain through a defect in the _____.

---

cranioplasty[27]

4. Use -plasty to write a term that means plastic surgery or surgical repair of the skull: _____

---

incision

5. Cranio/tomy[28] is _____ through the cranium or skull.

---

craniectomy[29]

6. Use -ectomy to write a term that, when translated literally, means excision of the skull, but actually means excision of a segment of the skull: _____

---

clavicle

7. Thorax[30] is used in medicine to refer to the chest. The major bones of the thorax are the clavicle, scapulae[31] (plural of scapula), sternum, and ribs. Clavicular[32] is an adjective that pertains to the _____.

---

scapula

8. Scapul/ar[33] pertains to the _____.

---

ribs

9. Cost/al[34] refers to the _____.

---

[26] kra'ne o sēl
[27] kra'ne o plas"te
[28] kra"ne ot'o me
[29] kra"ne ek'to me
[30] tho'raks

[31] skap'u le
[32] klah vik'u lar
[33] skap'u lar
[34] kos'tal

sternal[35]	10. Use the suffix -al (pertaining to) to write a word that means pertaining to the breast bone: _____
below	11. Sub/sternal[36] indicates a location or position _____ the sternum.
sternal	12. Sternal punctures are sometimes made with a needle to obtain a sample of bone marrow, the soft material that fills the central cavities of bones. Bone marrow samplings can be examined for the presence of abnormal cells. Puncture of the sternum with a needle is called a _____ puncture.
	13. There are twelve pairs of ribs, each one joined to a vertebra posteriorly (at the back). The first seven pairs, called "true ribs," have a direct attachment to the sternum. The other five pairs, referred to as "false ribs," do not attach directly to the sternum (Fig. 5–2).
ribs	14. Inter/costal[37] means between the _____. Intercostal muscles lie between the ribs and draw adjacent ribs together to increase the volume of the chest when breathing.
below (under)	15. Sub/costal[38] means _____ a rib or the ribs.
sternum **ribs**	16. Sterno/costal[39] pertains to the _____ and the _____.
costectomy[40]	17. Write a word that means excision of a rib: _____
vertebra	18. Vertebro/costal[41] pertains to a rib and a _____.
rib **vertebra**	19. Costo/vertebral[42] also means pertaining to a _____ and a _____. (Not all words can be reversed, as in vertebrocostal and costovertebral, but you will learn to recognize terms in which this can be done.)

[35] ster′nal
[36] sub ster′nal
[37] in″ter kos′tal
[38] sub kos′tal
[39] ster″no kos′tal
[40] kos tek′to me
[41] ver″tĕ bro kos′tal
[42] kos″to ver′tĕ bral

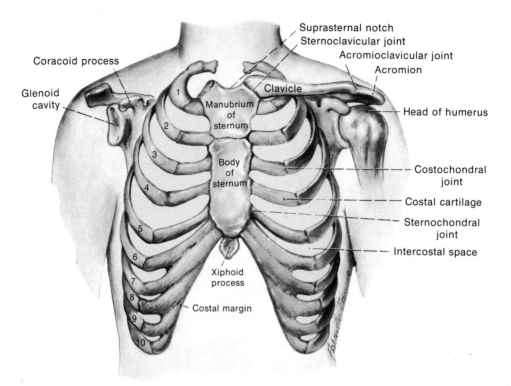

FIGURE 5-2

Anterior view of the rib cage. The ribs are found in pairs, one on each side of the chest, and are numbered from 1 to 12, beginning with the top rib. The upper seven pairs join directly with the sternum by a strip of cartilage and are called "true ribs." The remaining five pairs are referred to as "false ribs" because they do not attach directly to the sternum. The last two pairs of false ribs, the "floating ribs," are attached only on the posterior aspect. (From Jacob, S. W., Francone, C. A., and Lossow, W. J.: *Structure and Function in Man.* 5th ed. Philadelphia, W. B. Saunders, 1982.)

between	20. Inter/vertebral[43] means ＿＿＿＿＿＿＿ two adjoining ver-tebrae.[44]
· · · · · · · · · ·	21. Cushions of cartilage between adjoining vertebrae are called intervertebral disks. These layers of cartilage absorb shock. If they become diseased they sometimes rupture, resulting in a herniated[45] disk. This is commonly known as a slipped disk. If

[43] in"ter ver'tĕ bral
[44] ver'tĕ bre

[45] her'ne ăt"ed

herniated

vertebrae

spondylitis[47]

neck

chest

lower

thoracic, lumbar

bed rest does not alleviate the pain, surgery may be needed. The correct name for the rupture of an intervertebral disk is _____ disk.

22. Remembering that spondyl/o also means vertebra, spondylo/malacia[46] is softening of the _____.

23. Use spondyl/o to write a word that means inflammation of the vertebrae: _____

24. Thirty-three vertebrae comprise the spine, which is also called the spinal column or vertebral column. These bones enclose and protect the spinal cord, support the head, and serve as a place of attachment for the ribs and muscles of the back. The vertebrae are named and numbered from above downward (Fig. 5–3).

25. The combining form cervic/o means either neck or the cervix[48] of the uterus. In the naming of cervic/al vertebrae, cervical[49] refers to the _____. Figure 5–3 shows the seven cervical vertebrae, the C1 through C7 vertebrae.

26. The combining form thorac/o means the chest. Like other vertebrae, the thorac/ic vertebrae are so named because of their location, T1 through T12. The thoracic[50] vertebrae are part of the posterior (back) wall of the _____ cavity.

27. The combining form lumb/o means the lower back. Perhaps you have heard the word *lumbago*, which is a general term for a dull, aching pain in the lower back. The lumb/ar[51] vertebrae are located in the _____ back and are numbered L1 through L5.

28. Thoraco/lumbar[52] pertains to two types of vertebrae, the _____ and _____ vertebrae.

---

[46] spon"dĭ lo mah la'she ah
[47] spon"dĭ li'tis
[48] ser'viks
[49] ser'vĭ kal

[50] tho ras'ik
[51] lum'bar, lum'ber
[52] tho"rah ko lum'bar

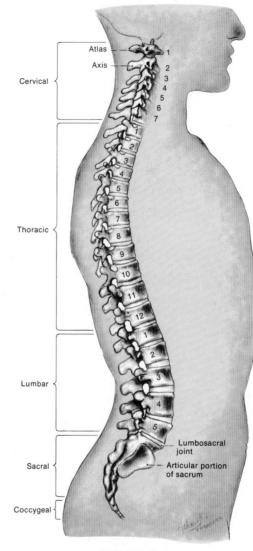

FIGURE 5–3

The vertebral column in relation to the body outline. The vertebrae are numbered from above downward. There are seven cervical vertebrae (C1 to C7) in the neck region, twelve thoracic vertebrae (T1 to T12) behind the chest cavity, five lumbar vertebrae (L1 to L5) supporting the lower back, five sacral vertebrae (S1 to S5) fused into one bone called the sacrum, and four coccygeal vertebrae (Co1 to Co4) fused into one bone called the coccyx. (From Jacob, S. W., Francone, C. A., and Lossow, W. J.: *Structure and Function in Man.* 5th ed. Philadelphia, W. B. Saunders, 1982.)

sacral

29. The combining form sacr/o refers to the sacrum, the triangular bone below the lumbar vertebrae. Five sacral[53] vertebrae are present at birth, but in the adult they are fused to form one bone. The sacrum is the result of fusion of five _____ bones.

coccygeal[54]

30. The coccyx is also the result of the fusion of vertebrae. The combining form coccyg/o means coccyx, or tail bone. This is located at the base of the spinal column and represents four fused coccyg/eal bones (-eal means pertaining to). The coccyx is the result of fusion of four _____ bones.

spine

31. The combining forms rach/i and rachi/o mean spine. Rachio/dynia[55] and rachi/algia[56] both mean painful _____.

pelvis

32. The lower vertebrae make up part of the pelvis, the basinlike structure formed by the sacrum, the coccyx, and the pelvic girdle (hip bones). The combining form pelv/i means pelvis. Pelv/ic[57] pertains to the_____.

ilium

33. The pelvic girdle consists of two hip bones. Each hip bone is three separate bones (ilium, ischium, and pubis) in the newborn, but these later fuse to form one bone in the adult. Ili/ac[58] pertains to the _____.

ischium

34. Ischi/al[59] pertains to the _____.

pubis

35. Pub/ic[60] pertains to the _____, located at the front of the pelvic girdle.

**ilium
pubis**

36. Ilio/pubic[61] pertains to the _____ and the _____.

---

[53] sa'kral
[54] kok sij'e al
[55] ra"ke o din'e ah
[56] ra"ke al'je ah
[57] pel'vik

[58] il'e ak
[59] is'ke al
[60] pu'bik
[61] il"e o pu'bik

ischiopubic[62]

ischiococcygeal[63]

humerus

ulna

ulnar[66]

humerus

radial[68]

carpectomy[69]

next

wrist
fingers

37. Use iliopubic as a model to write a word that means pertaining to the ischium and the pubis: _____

38. Use ischiopubic as a model to write a new term that means pertaining to the ischium and the coccyx: _____

39. Now practice using the word parts you have learned for the bones of the arm and hand. Humero/scapular[64] pertains to the _____ and the scapula.

40. Humero/ulnar[65] pertains to both the humerus and the _____.

41. From the previous frame, you should now recognize the adjective that means pertaining to the ulna. It is _____.

42. Humeral[67] means pertaining to the _____.

43. Use humeral as a model to write an adjective that means pertaining to the radius: _____

44. The wrist, also known as the carpus, consists of eight small bones called the carpals. Write a word that means excision of one or more bones of the wrist: _____

45. The metacarpals are located between the carpals and the phalanges. The prefix meta- means change, or next in a series. Meta/carpals lie _____ to the carpals.

46. The distal (far) ends of the metacarpals join with the fingers. Carpo/phalang/eal[70] refers to the _____ and the _____.

---

[62] is″ke o pu′bik
[63] is″ke o kok sij′e al
[64] hu″mer o skap′u lar
[65] hu″mer o ul′nar
[66] ul′nar

[67] hu′mer al
[68] ra′de al
[69] kar pek′to me
[70] kar″po fah lan′je al

phalangitis[71]	47. There are two phalanges in the thumb and three phalanges in each of the other four fingers. Write a word that means inflammation of the bones of the fingers or toes: _____
leg	48. The femur is the longest and heaviest bone in the body. Femur is the name of the bone of the upper _____.
femur	49. Ischio/femoral[72] pertains to the ischium and the _____.
femoral[73]	50. From the previous frame, you should recognize the adjective that means pertaining to the femur. The word is _____.
kneecap	51. Patello/femoral[74] pertains to the patella, or _____, and to the femur.
tibia	52. Two bones comprise the lower leg. The tibia is larger than the fibula. Tibi/algia[75] is pain of the _____.
tarsus	53. The tarsus, or ankle, has seven bones. Tarso/ptosis[76] is prolapse of the _____, and is commonly called flatfoot.
next	54. The meta/tarsals lie _____ to the tarsals and also join with bones of the toes.
bone	55. The rigid nature of bone gives it the ability to provide shape and support for the body. It is also important to remember, though, that bone contains living cells and is richly supplied with blood vessels and nerves. The combining form oste/o means bone. Oste/oid[77] means resembling _____.
osteitis[78]	56. Inflammation of a bone is _____.

---

[71] fal″an ji′tis
[72] is″ke o fem′o ral, is″ke o fem′or al
[73] fem′or al
[74] pah tel″o fem′o ral
[75] tib″e al′je ah
[76] tahr″sop to′sis
[77] os′te oid
[78] os″te i′tis

softness

57. Osteo/malacia[79] is a skeletal disorder characterized by a disturbance in bone metabolism. Remembering the meaning of -malacia, we know that osteo/malacia also means abnormal _____ of the bone.

calcium

58. The most common cause of osteomalacia is a deficiency of vitamin D. This vitamin is necessary for proper absorption of calcium, so a deficiency of vitamin D results in a shortage of _____, which is needed for bone growth and maintenance.

inflammation of the spine

bone

59. Insufficient calcium or vitamin D in children, during the growing years, causes rachitis, also called rickets. Rach/itis means _____.

Insufficient calcium in adults can lead to osteomalacia and osteoporosis.[80] The latter is seen most often in the elderly. Osteo/porosis means increased porosity of _____. The bones appear to be full of holes as a result of the deficiency of calcium.

calcium

60. The combining form calc/i means calcium. Calcification[81] is the process by which organic tissue becomes hardened by deposits of _____. Calcification in soft tissue is abnormal (e.g., deposition of calcium in the walls of arteries leads to arteriosclerosis).

calcium

61. De/calcification[82] is loss of _____ from bone or teeth. (The prefix de- means down, from, or reversing.)

softening

62. Osteomalacia is a consequence of decalcification without replacement of the lost calcium. Osteo/malacia is _____ of the bones.

63. Bone marrow is the soft organic material that fills the central cavity of a bone. The combining form for bone marrow is myel/o, which also refers to the spinal cord. It is sometimes difficult to know which meaning is intended. When you see myel/o you will

[79] os"te o mah la'she ah
[80] os"te o po ro'sis
[81] kal"sĭ fĭ ka'shun
[82] de"kal sĭ fĭ ka'shun

spinal cord **bone marrow**	need to decide if it means _____ _____ or _____ _____ .
inflammation	64. Myel/itis[83] means _____ of either the spinal cord or the bone marrow.
fiber (or fibrous)	65. Myelo/fibr/osis[84] is replacement of bone marrow by what type of tissue? _____
bone marrow	66. Osteo/myelitis[85] means inflammation of bone, especially of the _____ _____ .
spinal cord	67. Remembering that encephal/o means brain, myelo/encephal/ itis[86] means inflammation of the brain and _____ _____ .
	68. Congratulations if you knew which meaning was intended by *myel/o* in the last two frames! Its meaning is not always apparent, but you will be able to determine which meaning is intended through usage of the terms.

Some new word parts were introduced in the programmed learning that you have just completed. They are presented in the following list. Be sure that you **recognize their meanings.**

ADDITIONAL WORD PARTS AND THEIR MEANINGS

Word Part	Meaning
de-	down, from, or reversing
calc/i	calcium
cervic/o	neck or uterine cervix
coccyg/o	coccyx
lumb/o	lumbar

[83] mi"ĕ li'tis

[84] mi"ĕ lo fi bro'sis

[85] os"te o mi ĕ li'tis

[86] mi"ĕ lo en sef"ah li'tis

ADDITIONAL WORD PARTS AND THEIR MEANINGS (Continued)

Word Part	Meaning
myel/o	bone marrow or spinal cord
oste /o	bone
pelv/i	pelvis
rach/i, rachi/o	spine
sacr/o	sacrum
thorac/o	thorax (chest)

THE SPINE

Even though the vertebral column is composed of several bones it is still, in effect, a strong, flexible rod that moves anteriorly (forward), posteriorly (backward), and laterally (from side to side). Injury, disease, or other disorders of the spine have a significant influence on patients' ability to care for themelves. Some of the more important disorders will be presented here.

Injury to the Spine

In injuries of the spine, the greatest danger comes from the possibility that the spinal cord may be injured by movement of a fractured vertebra. Cord injury can cause paralysis below the point of injury. **Paraplegia**[87] is paralysis of the lower portion of the body and of both legs. (Not only injury, but also disease of the spinal cord, such as a tumor, can cause paralysis.) **Quadriplegia**[88] is paralysis of the arms and legs. (The prefix quadri- refers to all four extremities, both arms and both legs.)

    A **herniated disk** can press on the spinal cord or on a spinal nerve, causing pain. If bed rest does not relieve pain, a laminectomy[89] might be necessary. The lamina is the flattened part of either side of the arch of a vertebra. A **laminectomy** is excision of the posterior arch of a vertebra. When several disks are involved, spinal fusion may be done to immobilize the vertebrae.

Malformations of the Spine

Some spinal malformations are congenital and others can result from postural or nutritional defects or injury. **Spina bifida**[90] is a congenital abnormality characterized by defective closure of the bones of the

---

[87] par ah ple'je ah
[88] kwod"ri ple'je ah
[89] lam"ĭ nek'to me
[90] spi'nah bif'ĭ dah

spine. It can be so extensive that it allows herniation of the spinal cord, or it might be evident only on radiologic examination.

Scoliosis[91] is lateral curvature of the spine. It may be congenital but can also be caused by other conditions, such as hip disease. Exaggerated curvature of the spine from front to back gives rise to a condition called **kyphosis,**[92] commonly known as humpback or hunchback. It can result from congenital disorders or from certain diseases, but it is also seen in osteoporosis affecting the spine, particularly in women who suffer from calcium deficiency after menopause. It is believed that ingestion of sufficient calcium can prevent this latter problem.

Other Spinal Disorders

Rheumatoid spondylitis[93] causes inflammation of cartilage between the vertebrae, and can eventually cause neighboring vertebrae to fuse together. Sometimes the whole spine becomes stiffened, a condition called poker spine or **ankylosed**[94] **spine** (ankyl/o means stiff). Loss of spinal flexibility can also be caused by **osteoarthritis,**[95] a chronic disease involving the bones and joints, especially those joints that bear weight.

Other Terms Related to the Spine

Spinal anesthesia is loss of feeling produced by an anesthetic injected into the spinal canal. **Spinal puncture** (also called spinal tap or lumbar puncture) is puncture of the spinal cavity with a needle to extract the spinal fluid for diagnostic purposes, or to introduce agents into the spinal canal for anesthesia or radiographic studies. The **spinal cord** is part of the central nervous system. It is a cylindrical structure located in the spinal canal, extending from the lower part of the brain to the upper part of the lumbar region. **Spinal fluid** or **cerebrospinal**[96] **fluid** is the clear, colorless fluid that circulates throughout the brain and spinal cord.

CARTILAGE

Cartilage is a specialized type of dense connective tissue that is elastic but strong, and that can withstand considerable pressure or tension. Cartilage forms the major portion of the embryonic skeleton, but generally it is replaced by bone as the embryo matures. Cartilage does remain after birth, however, in the external ear, the nasal septum, the

---

91 sko"le o'sis
92 ki fo'sis
93 roo'mah toid spon"dĭ li'tis

94 ang'kĭ lōsd
95 os"te o ar thri'tis
96 ser"ĕ bro spi'nal

windpipe, between the vertebrae, and as a covering of bone surfaces at the places where they meet. The combining form for cartilage is chondr/o.

EXERCISE III

Using chondr/o (meaning cartilage) and other word parts you have learned, complete the sentences.

1. Chondr/al means pertaining to _____.
2. Vertebro/chondral refers to the vertebrae and the adjacent _____.
3. Chondro/costal pertains to the _____ and their associated _____.
4. Osteo/chondr/itis means inflammation of _____ and _____.
5. Sub/chondral means beneath the _____.
6. Surgical excision of diseased or damaged cartilage is _____.

(Check your answers.)

ARTICULATIONS AND ASSOCIATED STRUCTURES

The place of union between two or more bones is called an **articulation,**[97] or joint. Cartilage or other tissue covers the articular surface of bones. Joints that have cavities between articulating bones are called **synovial**[98] **joints.** This type of joint is freely movable and contains **synovial fluid.** The elbow, knee, ankle, shoulder, and hip joints are a few examples of synovial joints.

Movement tends to create friction between a bone and adjacent structures. **Bursae**[99] (plural of bursa) are sacs of fluid located in areas of friction, especially in the joints. **Burs/itis** is inflammation of a bursa (burs/o means bursa).

The combining form arthr/o means joint. You have probably heard of **arthritis,**[100] which is inflammation of a joint. **Rheumatoid arthritis** is a chronic disease characterized by inflammatory changes in joints and related structures, and can result in crippling deformities. (**Rheumatism**[101] is a general term for acute and chronic conditions characterized by inflammation, soreness, and stiffness of muscles, and by pain in joints and associated structures.) There are many

---

[97] ar tik"u la'shun
[98] sĭ no've al
[99] ber'se

[100] ar thri'tis
[101] roo'mah tizm

other types of arthritis, including osteoarthritis (mentioned above) and spondylarthritis.[102] **Spondyl/arthritis** means inflammation of a vertebra, or it can be thought of as arthritis of the spine. (For easier pronunciation the *o* is dropped from spondyl/o when joined with arthritis.) **Polyarthritis**[103] means inflammation of more than one joint (poly- means many). Both **arthralgia**[104] and **arthrodynia**[105] mean painful joint. **Arthro/centesis**[106] is needle puncture of a joint space, usually done to remove excess fluid that has accumulated.

The knee, a synovial joint, is subject to many injuries, including dislocation, sprain, and fracture. The most common injury is tearing of the cartilage. **Arthroscopy**[107] is direct visualization of the interior of a joint. The procedure uses a fiberoptic instrument called an **arthroscope,**[108] and requires only a few small incisions. Bits of diseased or damaged cartilage can be removed during this procedure. Incision of a joint is **arthrotomy.**[109] **Arthropathy**[110] means any disease of a joint. **Ankylosis**[111] (ankyl/o means stiff) is an abnormal condition in which the joint is immobile and stiff.

Ligaments are strong bands of fibrous connective tissue that connect bones or cartilages, and serve to support and strengthen joints. Ligamentous means related to or like a ligament.

MUSCLES AND ASSOCIATED STRUCTURES

Muscle is composed of cells or fibers that contract and bring about movement of an organ or part of the body. There are three main types of muscle tissue: cardiac (heart) muscle, smooth muscle (found in the internal organs), and skeletal muscle, which is under conscious or voluntary control. The muscular system, however, usually refers only to skeletal muscle. The term **fascia**[112] is used for the fibrous membrane that covers, supports, and separates muscles. **Tendons** are bands of strong fibrous tissue that attach the muscles to the bones. The combining forms ten/o and tend/o mean tendon. Tendons can become damaged if a wound is deep. **Tendoplasty**[113] is surgical repair of a tendon. **Tendonitis**[114] means inflammation of a tendon. Notice that the combining form is not used in writing the term tendonitis.

---

[102] spon"dil ar thri'tis
[103] pol"e ar thri'tis
[104] ar thral'je ah
[105] ar"thro din'e ah
[106] ar"thro sen te'sis
[107] ar thros'ko pe
[108] ar'thro skōp
[109] ar throt'o me
[110] ar throp'ah the
[111] ang"kĭ lo'sis
[112] fash'e ah
[113] ten'do plas"te
[114] ten"do ni'tis

EXERCISE IV   *Two combining forms that mean muscle are muscul/o and my/o. Using these combining forms and other word parts you have learned, write words in the blanks to complete the sentences. This exercise teaches you several new terms and is not a review.*

1. Teno/myo/plasty[115] is surgical repair of tendon and
   _____ .

2. Use my/o to write a term that means destruction of muscle:
   _____

3. Myo/cellul/itis[116] is inflammation of cellular tissue and
   _____ .

4. Use my/o to write a word that means any disease of muscle:
   _____

5. Myo/fibr/osis[117] is a condition in which _____ tissue is replaced by fibrous tissue. (Remember that fibr/o means fiber.)

6. A myo/cele[118] is a condition in which _____ protrudes through its fascial covering. This is also called a fascial hernia. Fascial[119] pertains to the fascia.

7. Musculo/fascial[120] pertains to or consists of _____ and fascia.

8. Progressive muscul/ar dystrophy is a familial disease characterized by progressive wasting of _____ .

9. My/asthenia (-asthenia means weakness) is muscular weakness. Myasthenia gravis[121] is a disease of unknown cause characterized by great _____ weakness.

10. My/algia[122] is muscle _____ .

(Check your answers.)

Several more combining forms have been introduced in this chapter. They are presented in the following list.

ADDITIONAL COMBINING FORMS AND THEIR MEANINGS

Combining Form	Meaning
ankyl/o	stiff
arthr/o	articulation, joint

---

[115] ten″o mi′o plas″te
[116] mi″o sel″u li′tis
[117] mi″o fi bro′sis
[118] mi′o sēl

[119] fash′e al
[120] mus″ku lo fash′e al
[121] mi″as the′ne ah grav′is
[122] mi al′je ah

ADDITIONAL COMBINING FORMS AND THEIR MEANINGS (Continued)

Combining Form	Meaning
burs/o	bursa
chondr/o	cartilage
muscul/o, my/o	muscle
ten/o, tend/o	tendon

DISEASES, DISORDERS, AND DIAGNOSTIC TERMS

Collagen[123] **diseases** are a group of diseases of the connective tissue. Collagen is a fibrous protein of connective tissue. Generalized inflammation of the connective tissue and blood vessels is usually seen in collagen disease. The cause is unknown. **Lupus erythematosus**[124] (LE) and **scleroderma**[125] (scler/o, dry, + derm/a, skin) are collagen diseases. *Lupus* is Latin for wolf; the disease was so named because of a characteristic rash across the nose in some patients.

A **dislocation** is displacement of a bone from a joint.

Fracture is the sudden breaking of a bone, usually resulting from injury. Bones sometimes break spontaneously, though, as in osteomalacia, osteomyelitis, and certain other conditions or diseases. In a **simple fracture** the bone is broken but does not puncture the skin surface. The broken bone is visible through an opening in the skin when a **compound fracture** has occurred. If the bone is no longer in alignment it is treated by **reduction,** which pulls the broken ends into alignment. If a fractured bone is restored to its normal position by manipulation without surgery, it is a **closed reduction.** If the fractured bone must be exposed by surgery, it is an **open reduction.** Sometimes **internal fixation** is necessary, in which a rod or plate is inserted to stabilize the bone's alignment.

Gout is a painful metabolic disease that is a form of acute arthritis. It is characterized by inflammation of the joints, especially of those in the foot or knee. It is hereditary and results from **hyperuricemia**[126] (hyper, excessive, + uric, which refers to uric acid, + -emia, blood) and from deposits of urates in and around joints.

A **hernia** is protrusion of an organ or part of an organ through the wall of the cavity that normally contains it. Certain areas of the abdominal wall tend to be weak spots, and hernias are more likely to occur in such places. Inguinal hernias,[127] accounting for about 80% of all hernias, are caused by rupture or separation of a portion of the

---

[123] kol′ah jen
[124] loo′pus er″ĭ the″mah to′sis
[125] skle″ro der′mah

[126] hi″per u″rĭ se′me ah
[127] ing′gwi nal her′ne ahz

abdominal wall. This results in the protrusion of a hernial sac containing part of the intestine.

Leukemias[128] are chronic or acute diseases of the blood-forming tissues characterized by unrestrained growth of leukocytes and their precursors. Bone marrow is important in blood production and is involved in some types of leukemia. Leukemias are classified according to the dominant cell type and severity of the disease.

Multiple myeloma[129] (myel/o, bone marrow, + -oma, tumor) is a disease characterized by the presence of many tumor masses in the bone and bone marrow. It is usually progressive and generally fatal.

Osteitis deformans[130] (Paget's disease) is a skeletal disease of the elderly characterized by chronic bone inflammation. This results in thickening and softening of bones and in bowing of the long bones.

The **sarcomas**[131] are cancers that arise from connective tissue, such as muscle or bone. A **chondrosarcoma**[132] is composed of masses of cartilage. A **fibrosarcoma**[133] is a malignant tumor containing much fibrous tissue.

A **sprain** is injury to a joint that causes pain and disability, depending on the degree of injury to ligaments or tendons.

A **strain** is excessive use of a part of the body to the extent that it is injured, or trauma to a muscle caused by violent contraction or excessive forcible stretch.

EXERCISE V

Match the terms in the left column with their meanings in the right column.

_____ 1. compound fracture
_____ 2. dislocation
_____ 3. hernia
_____ 4. reduction
_____ 5. simple fracture
_____ 6. strain

A. muscle trauma or injury caused by excessive use of the body part
B. bone is broken, but does not protrude through the skin
C. bone is broken and protrudes through an opening in the skin
D. displacement of a bone from a joint
E. pulling the broken ends of a bone into alignment
F. protrusion of an organ through the wall of the cavity that normally contains it

---

[128] loo ke'me ahz
[129] mi ĕ lo'mah
[130] os"te i'tis de for'manz
[131] sar ko'mahz
[132] kon"dro sar ko'mah
[133] fi"bro sar ko'mah

EXERCISE VI

Match the terms in the left column with their meanings in the right column (not all selections will be used).

_____ 1. gout
_____ 2. leukemia
_____ 3. multiple mye-
      loma
_____ 4. sarcoma

A. unrestrained growth of leukocytes and their precursors
B. cancer that arises from connective tissue
C. a large group of diseases of which lupus erythematosus is an example
D. a skeletal disease of the elderly with chronic inflammation of bones
E. characterized by many tumor masses in the bone and bone marrow
F. marked by inflammation of the joints, resulting from hyperuricemia

Comprehensive Review Exercises

WORK THE FOLLOWING EXERCISES TO TEST YOUR UNDERSTANDING OF THE MATERIAL IN CHAPTER 5. IT IS BEST TO DO ALL THE REVIEW EXERCISES BEFORE CHECKING YOUR ANSWERS.

A. Write a word or word part in each blank to complete the table. Common names are given. The first one has been done as an example.

Common Name	Scientific Name	Combining Form
1. wrist	carpus	carp/o
2. collarbone	_____	_____
3. skull	_____	_____
4. thigh bone	_____	_____
5. kneecap	_____	_____
6. shoulder blade	_____	_____
7. breastbone	_____	_____
8. ankle	_____	_____

B. There are five types of vertebrae. Write the name of a type of vertebrae to complete each sentence.

1. C1 through C7 are _____ vertebrae.

2. T1 through T12 are _____ vertebrae.

3. L1 through L5 are _____ vertebrae.

4. Five _____ vertebrae are fused into one bone, called the sacrum.

5. Four _____ vertebrae are fused into one bone, called the coccyx.

C. Four terms are given in each of the following. Three of the terms have a great deal in common, but one is not consistent with the other three. Find the *inconsistent* term in each of the following and circle it.

1. costa, humerus, radius, ulna
2. iliac, ischial, phalangeal, pubic
3. carpal, femur, fibula, tibia
4. clavicular, cranial, scapular, sternal
5. osteoarthritis, hematopoiesis, polyarthritis, rheumatism

D. Match the underlined word parts in the left column with their meanings in the right column (some answers will be used more than once).

_____ 1. thoraco<u>lumb</u>ar	A. calcium
_____ 2. <u>rachi</u>algia	B. ilium
_____ 3. <u>teno</u>myoplasty	C. ischium
_____ 4. <u>myo</u>cellulitis	D. joint
_____ 5. my<u>asthenia</u>	E. lower back
_____ 6. <u>cervic</u>al vertebrae	F. muscle
	G. neck
_____ 7. <u>calci</u>fication	H. spine
_____ 8. <u>ilio</u>pubic	I. stiff
_____ 9. <u>arthr</u>algia	J. tendon
_____ 10. <u>tendo</u>plasty	K. weakness
_____ 11. <u>ankyl</u>osis	L. vertebra
_____ 12. <u>spondyl</u>itis	

E. Using word parts you have learned, write letters in the blanks to complete each sentence.

1. Excision of a portion of the skull is __ __ __ __ __ectomy.

2. Inter __ __ __ __ __ __ muscles lie between the ribs.

3. The tail bone is also called the __ __ __ __ __ __.

4. Softening of the vertebrae is __ __ __ __ __ __ __ __mala-cia.

5. Rupture of an intervertebral disk is also called __ __ __ __ __ __ __ __ __ disk.

6. Pertaining to the wrist and the fingers is __ __ __ __ __—phalangeal.

7. Prolapse of the ankle is __ __ __ __ __—ptosis.

8. Resembling bone is __ __ __ __—oid.

9. Replacement of bone marrow by fibrous tissue is __ __ __ __ __—fibrosis.

10. A chronic disease involving the bones and joints is osteo __ __ __ __ __—itis.

F. Circle the correct answer to complete each sentence.

1. Lateral curvature of the spine is (kyphosis, rickets, scoliosis, spina bifida).

2. Inflammation of the bone, especially of the bone marrow, is (osteitis deformans, osteomalacia, osteoporosis, osteomyelitis).

3. Excision of cartilage is (chondrectomy, chondrocostal, subchondral, vertebrochondral).

4. Articulation is another name for (fascia, joint, ligament, tendon).

5. Sacs of fluid located in areas of friction, especially in the joints, are called (bursae, fasciae, laminae, septa).

6. Inflammation of more than one joint is (arthrocentesis, arthrodynia, polyarthritis, quadriplegia.)

7. Displacement of a bone from a joint is called (dislocation, fracture, sprain, strain).

8. Pulling the broken ends of a bone into alignment by manipulation without surgery is called (closed reduction, compound fracture, open reduction, simple fracture).

9. A weakness in the abdominal wall resulting in protrusion of a hernial sac containing part of the intestine is called (inguinal hernia, multiple myeloma, myocele, polymyositis).

10. A malignant tumor composed of cartilage is (chondrosarcoma, gout, leukemia, sarcoidosis).

G. Write the medical term for which each meaning is given.

1. surgical repair of the skull _____

2. excision of a rib _____

3. visualization of the interior of a joint _____

4. inflammation of a joint _____

5. incision of the cranium _____

6. below the breastbone_____

7. pertaining to a rib and vertebra _____ or _____.

8. branch of medicine that specializes in the skeletal and muscular systems _____

The Circulatory System

OBJECTIVES

After completing Chapter 6, you will be able to

1. Write and select the correct meaning of each word part.
2. Recognize the cardiovascular and lymphatic systems as parts of the circulatory system.
3. Write terms when presented with their definitions and select the appropriate response when presented with several answers.
4. Match diseases, disorders, and diagnostic terms pertaining to the circulatory system with their descriptions.

OUTLINE

STRUCTURE AND FUNCTION OF THE CIRCULATORY SYSTEM
THE HEART
    Diseases, Disorders, and Diagnostic Terms Pertaining to the Heart
    Diagnosis and Treatment of Heart Disease
BLOOD VESSELS
THE BLOOD
THE LYMPHATIC SYSTEM
COMPREHENSIVE REVIEW EXERCISES

STRUCTURE AND FUNCTION OF THE CIRCULATORY SYSTEM

The **circulatory system** consists of the **cardiovascular**[1] system (heart and blood vessels) and the **lymphatic**[2] system (structures involved in the conveyance of the fluid **lymph**[3]). The term **cardiovascular** (cardi/o, heart, and vas/o, vessel) pertains to the heart and blood vessels. Adequate functioning of the circulatory system is essential for **homeostasis**,[4] equilibrium of the internal environment of the body. Homeostasis is derived from home/o, meaning sameness, and -stasis, meaning constant. When homeostasis is disrupted, ill health and even death may result. Homeostasis is maintained by intricate relationships between the body systems.

Body cells must have a constant supply of food, oxygen, and other substances to function properly. Fluid outside body cells is called **extracellular**[5] **fluid** (extra- means outside). This fluid is found principally in two places. In blood vessels extracellular fluid is called **plasma**.[6] Fluid that fills spaces between cells outside the blood vessels is called **intercellular**,[7] **interstitial**,[8] or **tissue fluid**. Fluid located inside cells is **intracellular**[9] **fluid** (intra- means within).

The cardiovascular system supplies body cells with needed substances and transports waste products for disposal. Label Figure 6–1 as you read the accompanying paragraphs.

THE HEART

The heart is a muscular pump that circulates the blood. It is enclosed in a sac made up of a double membrane called the **pericardium**[10] (peri-, around, + cardi/o, heart, + -ium, membrane). Notice that one i is dropped when cardi/o and -ium are joined (this is done to facilitate pronunciation). Inflammation of the pericardium is **pericarditis**[11] (-itis, inflammation). This can be caused by infectious microorganisms or a cancerous growth, or it can have various other causes. Another membrane, the **endocardium**[12] (endo-, inside), forms the lining inside the heart. **Endocarditis**[13] is often caused by infective microorganisms that invade the endocardium. The valves of the heart are frequently affected in endocarditis. The heart muscle itself is called the **myocardium**[14] (my/o, muscle). This is the thickest tissue of the heart and is composed of muscle fibers that contract, resulting in the squeezing of blood from the heart with each heartbeat. **Myo-**

---

[1] kar″de o vas′ku lar
[2] lim fat′ik
[3] limf
[4] ho″me o sta′sis
[5] eks″trah sel′u lar
[6] plaz′mah
[7] in″ter sel′u lar
[8] in″ter stish′al
[9] in″trah sel′u lar
[10] per″ĭ kar′de um
[11] per″ĭ kar di′tis
[12] en″do kar′de um
[13] en″do kar di′tis
[14] mi″o kar′de um

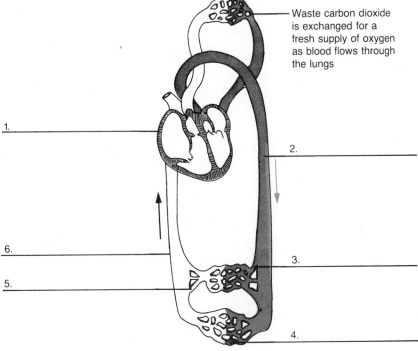

Waste carbon dioxide
is exchanged for a
fresh supply of oxygen
as blood flows through
the lungs

1.

2.

6.

5.

3.

4.

FIGURE 6–1

The circulatory system. Label the drawing as you read. Blood that is rich in oxygen is pumped by the heart *(1)* to all parts of the body. It leaves the heart by the arteries *(2)*, which branch many times and become arterioles *(3)*. The arterioles branch out even more to become one-cell-thick vessels called capillaries *(4)*. In the capillaries oxygen is released and waste carbon dioxide is collected. Blood leaving the capillaries returns to the heart through the venules *(5)*, which flow into the veins *(6)*. The veins carry the blood back to the heart. Before it is once again pumped to the body cells it picks up a fresh supply of oxygen by passing through the lungs. (From Leonard, P. C.: *Building a Medical Vocabulary*. 2nd ed. Philadelphia, W. B. Saunders, 1988.)

carditis[15] is inflammation of the heart muscle, and is one example of a **cardiomyopathy**[16] (cardi/o, heart, + my/o, muscle, + -pathy, disease). Cardiomyopathy is a general diagnostic term that designates primary heart disease.

Blood vessels that supply oxygen to the heart are **coronary arteries.** Coronary[17] means encircling, in the manner of a crown, and refers to the way in which coronary arteries encircle the heart in a

---

[15] mi″o kar di′tis   [17] kor′ŏ na re
[16] kar″de o mi op′ah the

crownlike fashion. Coronary heart disease (CHD), heart damage resulting from insufficient oxygen, is caused by pathologic changes in the coronary arteries.

Blood pressure is the pressure exerted by the blood on the wall of an artery. Indirect blood pressure readings generally consist of two numbers expressed as a fraction. A healthy young person has a blood pressure of approximately 120/80. The first number is higher than the second and represents the maximum pressure on the artery. The second number is the amount of pressure that still exists when the heart is relaxed (in other words, not contracting). Elevated blood pressure is called **hypertension**[18] (hyper-, excessive, or above normal). Usually, if the first number is consistently above 140 mm of mercury or the second number is consistently above 100, the person is considered to have hypertension. Low blood pressure is known as **hypotension**[19] (hypo-, below normal). A blood pressure of 95/60 indicates hypotension, but each person's reading must be interpreted individually.

Diseases, Disorders, and Diagnostic Terms Pertaining to the Heart

angina pectoris[20] severe pain and constriction about the heart caused by an insufficient supply of blood to the heart itself. (Angina is derived from a Latin word that means to choke. Angina is frequently used with other terms, and refers to pain of that particular part. Pectoris refers to the chest, and is derived from the Latin *pectora*, chest.)

arrhythmia[21] (a-, without): irregularity or loss of rhythm of the heartbeat

cardiomegaly[22] (cardi/o, heart, + -megaly, enlargement): enlarged size of the heart

congenital heart defects: abnormalities present in the heart at birth (congenital means existing at birth). These defects often involve the septum, a partition that divides the right and left chambers of the heart.

fibrillation[23]: a severe cardiac arrhythmia in which contractions are too rapid and uncoordinated for effective blood circulation. It can sometimes be reversed by the use of a **defibrillator,**[24] an electronic apparatus that delivers a shock to the heart, often through the placement of electrodes on the chest (de- means down, from, or reversing). **De/fibrillation**[25] reverses fibrillation. Defibrillation is the same as cardioversion.[26]

heart failure: cessation of the heartbeat; a clinical condition resulting from failure of the heart to pump the blood effectively and to maintain adequate circulation of the blood.

congestive heart failure (CHF): a condition characterized by weakness, breathlessness, and edema[27] (swelling caused by excessive tissue

---

[18] hi"per ten'shun
[19] hi"po ten'shun
[20] an ji'nah or an'ji nah pek'to res
[21] ah rith'me ah
[22] kar"de o meg'ah le

[23] fi brĭ la'shun, fi bril a'shun
[24] de fib"rĭ la'tor
[25] de fib'rĭ la'shun
[26] kar de o ver'zhun
[27] ĕ de'mah

fluid) in lower portions of the body—the work demanded of the heart is greater than its ability to perform.

heart murmur: a soft blowing or rasping sound that may be heard when listening to the heart, not necessarily pathologic

hyperlipemia[28] (hyper-, excessive, + lip/o, fat, + -emia, blood): an excessive quantity of fat in the blood

infarction[29]: formation of a localized area of tissue that undergoes necrosis[30] following lack of blood supply to that area. Necrosis is death of tissue. It can result from **occlusion**[31] (obstruction) or **stenosis**[32] (narrowing) of the artery that supplies blood to that tissue. **Myocardial**[33] **infarction** (MI) is death of an area of the heart muscle that occurs as a result of oxygen deprivation (also called acute myocardial infarction, AMI).

myocardial ischemia: deficiency of blood supply to the myocardium (the word *ischemia*[34] refers to temporary deficiency of blood supply to any body part).

shock: a serious condition in which blood flow to the heart is reduced to such an extent that body tissues do not receive enough blood. This condition can result in death. Shock may have various causes, including hemorrhage, infection, drug reaction, injury, poisoning, MI, and excessive emotional stress.

Diagnosis and Treatment of Heart Disorders

Major advances have recently been made in treating heart disease, including heart transplantation, the replacement of a diseased heart using a donor organ. **Open heart surgery** refers to operative procedures on the heart after it has been exposed through incision of the chest wall. **Cardiopulmonary**[35] (heart-lung) **bypass** is the method used to divert blood away from the heart and lungs temporarily when surgery of the heart and major vessels is performed. A heart-lung pump collects the blood, replenishes it with oxygen, and returns it to the body. **Pulmonary** refers to the lungs (pulmon/o, lungs, + -ary, pertaining to). **Cardiopulmonary** means the heart and lungs.

The heart has a natural pacemaker called the sinoatrial[36] (SA) node. Often, however, when discussing a pacemaker in reference to the heart, an artificial pacemaker is implied. A **pacemaker implant** is an artificial pacemaker implanted to keep the heart rhythm within a desirable range in patients who suffer from severe arrhythmia. The electrodes that deliver the electrical impulses to the heart are placed either on the chest (an external pacemaker) or within the chest wall (an internal pacemaker).

Cardiac catheterization[37] is the passage of a long flexible tube into the heart chambers through a vein in an arm or leg, or the neck. Cardi/ac (cardi/o + -ac, pertaining to) refers to the heart. An instru-

---

[28] hi″per li pe′me ah
[29] in fark′shun
[30] ně kro′sis
[31] ŏ kloo′zhun
[32] stě no′sis

[33] mi″o kar′de al
[34] is ke′me ah
[35] kar″de o pul′mo ner e
[36] si″no a′tre al
[37] kar′de ak kath″ě ter i za′shun

ment called a **catheter**[38] is used. This allows the collection of blood samples from different parts of the heart and determines pressure differences in various chambers. Combined with special endoscopic (endo-, inside, + scop/o, to view, + -ic, pertaining to) equipment, cardiac catheterization allows internal parts of the heart to be viewed. An **endoscopic**[39] **examination** uses an **endoscope,**[40] a device consisting of a tube and optical system for observing inside a hollow organ or cavity.

Noninvasive procedures do not require entering the body or puncturing the skin, and therefore are less hazardous for the patient than invasive procedures. Several noninvasive procedures are available for the diagnosis of heart disease. Conventional x-ray procedures provide information about heart size and gross abnormalities, but newer methods have greatly contributed to information about the heart. **Ultrasound,** also called ultrasonography, uses sound waves bounced off tissue to produce a record called a **sonogram**[41] (son/o, sound, + -gram, a record). Echo- also means sound, and **echocardiography**[42] (-graphy, process of recording) is the term generally associated with the use of ultrasonography in diagnosing heart disease. The **echocardiogram**[43] is the record of the heart obtained by directing ultrasonic waves through the chest wall. **Computed tomography**[44] (CT) is another noninvasive diagnostic procedure. It produces cross-sectional images of an organ similar to what would be seen if the actual organ were cut into sections. CT was once known as computerized axial tomography (CAT), and the term CAT scan is still used; CT, however, is more commonly used. A diagnostic procedure that has been available longer than many of the others is **electrocardiography**[45] (electr/o, electricity). The record obtained, the **electrocardiogram** (ECG),[46] is produced by recording the electrical currents of the heart muscle using a device called an **electrocardiograph.**[47]

Cardiopulmonary resuscitation[48] (CPR) is recommended as an emergency first-aid procedure to re-establish heart and lung action if breathing or heart action has stopped. It consists of closed heart massage and artificial respiration. CPR provides basic life support until it is no longer needed or until more advanced life support equipment is available.

---

[38] kath'ĕ ter
[39] en do skop'ik
[40] en'do skōp
[41] so'no gram
[42] ek"o kar"de og'rah fe
[43] ek"o kar'de o gram"

[44] to mog'rah fe
[45] e lek"tro kar"de og'rah fe
[46] e lek"tro kar'de o gram"
[47] e lek"tro kar'de o graf"
[48] re sus ĭ ta'shun

EXERCISE I   Match the types of heart tissue in the left column with their meanings in the right column.

_____ 1. endocardium   A. the muscular middle layer of the
_____ 2. myocardium   heart
_____ 3. pericardium   B. the lining of the heart
                         C. the sac that encloses the heart

(Check your answers with the solutions in the back of the book.)

EXERCISE II   Match the following diseases, disorders, or diagnostic terms pertaining to the heart in the left column with their meanings in the right column.

_____ 1. angina pectoris   A. death of an area of the heart muscle
_____ 2. cardiomegaly   B. abnormality present in the heart at
_____ 3. cardiomyopa-   birth
         thy   C. soft blowing or rasping heart sound
_____ 4. congenital   D. contractions that are too rapid and
         heart defect   uncoordinated for effective blood
_____ 5. congestive   circulation
         heart failure   E. elevated blood pressure
_____ 6. fibrillation   F. severe pain and constriction about
_____ 7. heart murmur   the heart caused by insufficient
_____ 8. myocardial   blood supply
         infarction   G. condition characterized by weak-
_____ 9. myocardial   ness, shortness of breath, and
         ischemia   edema of the lower portions of the
_____ 10. hypertension   body
                             H. deficiency of blood supply to the
                                heart
                             I. general designation for primary
                                myocardial disease
                             J. enlarged heart

EXERCISE III   Using words and word parts you have learned, write letters in the blanks to complete each sentence.

1. A severe cardiac arrhythmia in which contractions are uncoordinated and ineffective, which can sometimes be reversed by using a defibrillator, is called f __ __ __ __ __ __ __ __ __ __ __.

2. An excessive quantity of fat in the blood is hyper- __ __ __ __ __ __.

3. Referring to the lungs and heart is __ __ __ __ __ __—pulmo-nary.

4. A device consisting of a tube and optical system that is used to observe inside a hollow organ or cavity is called an endo- __ __ __ __ __.

5. An electrical device that can keep the heart rhythm within a desirable range is a cardiac __ __ __ __ __ __ __ __ __.

EXERCISE IV

Match the medical terms in the left column with their meanings in the right column.

____ 1. cardiac cathe-terization

____ 2. cardiopulmo-nary bypass

____ 3. cardiopulmo-nary resuscita-tion

____ 4. computed tomography

____ 5. echocardiogra-phy

____ 6. electrocardio-gram

____ 7. sonogram

A. use of ultrasound in the diagnosis of heart disease

B. record produced in ultrasonography

C. passage of a long flexible tube into the heart chambers through a vein

D. method used to divert blood away from the heart and lungs during heart surgery

E. diagnostic procedure that produces images of organ cross sections

F. emergency first-aid procedure used to re-establish heart and lung action

G. record produced by recording the electrical currents of the heart muscle

(Check your answers.)

BLOOD VESSELS

Five types of blood vessels are shown in Figure 6–1: **arteries,** smaller arteries called **arterioles,**[49] **veins,** smaller veins called **venules,**[50] and **capillaries.**[51] You already know that vas/o and angi/o are combining forms that mean vessel, in general. Angio/card/itis[52] is inflammation of the heart and large vessels. (Angiocarditis is derived from angi/o, vessel, + cardi/o, heart, + -itis, inflammation. Notice that one *i* is dropped to avoid the use of a double *i* and to make pronunciation

---

[49] ar te′re ōlz
[50] ven′ūlz

[51] kap′ĭ lar′ez
[52] an″je o kar di′tis

easier.) The term **vascular**[53] pertains to blood vessels. **Vasodilation**[54] is an increase in the diameter of a blood vessel. **Vasoconstriction**[55] has the opposite meaning of vasodilation. The dilation and constriction of blood vessels influence blood pressure as well as distribution of blood to various parts of the body. **Vasodilators,**[56] drugs that dilate the blood vessels, are sometimes used to treat hypertension.

    Angiomas (angi/o, vessel, + -oma, tumor) are tumors consisting principally of blood vessels (**hemangioma**[57]) or lymph vessels (**lymphangioma**[58]). Such tumors are usually benign (not malignant). In the term hem/angi/oma, hem/a or hem/o means blood.

    Commit the meanings of the combining forms in the following table to **memory.**

COMBINING FORMS FOR SPECIFIC VESSELS

Combining Form	Meaning
aort/o	aorta[59]
arteri/o	artery
arteriol/o	arteriole
phleb/o, ven/o	vein
venul/o	venule

PROGRAMMED LEARNING

Remember to cover the answers in the left column. Slide the card down to check each answer after you write the answer in the blank.

arteriopathy[60]	1. Remembering that -pathy means disease, write a word that means any disease of the arteries: _____

---

[53] vas′ku lar
[54] vas″o di la′shun
[55] vas″o kon strik′shun
[56] vas″o di lāt′orz

[57] hĕ man″je o′mah
[58] lim fan″je o′mah
[59] a or′tah
[60] ar″te re op′ah the

artery

2. Arter/itis[61] is inflammation of an _____. (Notice that one *i* is omitted to make pronunciation easier.)

arteries

3. Arterio/scler/osis[62] is hardening of the _____.

4. Arteriosclerosis is a thickening and loss of elasticity of the walls of the arteries. This is a major cause of hypertension. Athero/sclerosis,[63] a form of arteriosclerosis, is characterized by the formation of fatty, cholesterol-like deposits on the walls of arteries. Ather/o means yellow, fatty plaque. Use ather/o to write the term that designates a form of arteriosclerosis:

atherosclerosis

_____

5. Arteries carry blood away from the heart. The aorta, the largest artery in the body, is about 3 cm in diameter at its origin in the left side of the heart. The aorta has many branches, and early divisions of this vessel supply the heart, head, and upper part of the body. The combining form for aorta is _____.

aort/o

6. Write a word that means inflammation of the aorta:

aortitis[64]

_____

7. Aorto/graphy[65] is radiography of the aorta after the injection of a solution to enhance the image of the aorta on x-ray. Write a word that means the film produced during aortography:

aortogram[66]

_____

8. Use angi/o to write a word that means radiography of the vessels, in general: _____

angiography[67]

9. Angio/cardio/graphy[68] is roentgenography[69] (radiography) of the _____ and great vessels after intravenous (intra-, within, + ven/o, vein) injection of a radiopaque[70] solu-

heart

---

[61] ar″tĕ ri′tis
[62] ar te″re o sklĕ ro′sis
[63] ath″er o″skle ro′sis
[64] a″or ti′tis
[65] a″or tog′rah fe

[66] a or′to gram″
[67] an″je og′rah fe
[68] an″je o kar″de og′rah fe
[69] rent″gen og′rah fe
[70] ra″de o pāk′

tion. Radi/o means radiant energy. Radiopaque means not permitting the passage of radiant energy, or opaque to radiant energy.

---

aorta

10. An aneurysm[71] is a ballooning out of the wall of a vessel, usually an artery, caused by a congenital defect or weakness of the wall of the vessel. Aortic[72] aneurysms can affect any part of which vessel? _____

---

aortoplasty[73]

11. A potentially dangerous effect of an aneurysm is rupture of the vessel and resulting hemorrhage. An aortic aneurysm can be repaired by surgery. Write a word that means surgical repair of the aorta: _____

---

vessel

12. In a cerebral aneurysm there is ballooning out of a blood _____ in the brain. Cerebr/al (cerebr/o + -al, pertaining to) refers to the cerebrum or brain. A dangerous effect of a cerebral aneurysm is cerebral hemorrhage.

---

cerebrovascular

13. Another dangerous effect of a cerebral aneurysm is a cerebro/vascular[74] accident (CVA). This is also called a stroke or stroke syndrome. CVA can also be caused by blood vessels that have become narrowed or blocked. CVA is the abbreviation for _____ accident.

---

arteries

14. The aorta branches out to form arteries. Arteri/al[75] means pertaining to one or more _____.

---

arteritis

15. Use -itis to write a term that means inflammation of an artery: _____

---

many

16. Poly/arter/itis[76] is a disease that involves inflammation of _____ arteries. It leads to diminished flow of blood to areas normally supplied by these arteries.

---

[71] an'u rizm
[72] a or'tik
[73] a ort'o plas"te

[74] ser"ĕ bro vas'ku lar
[75] ar te're al
[76] pol"e ar"tĕ ri'tis

polyarteritis

17. A disease that involves inflammation of several arteries is called
_____.

artery (arteries)

18. Arteries are used to measure the pulse rate. The pulse is the periodic thrust felt over the arteries that is consistent with the heartbeat. The pulse, the rhythmic expansion of the _____, can be felt with a finger.

bradycardia[78]

19. The normal pulse rate of an adult in a resting state is approximately 70 to 80 beats/minute. An increased pulse rate is called tachy/cardia[77] (tachy-, fast, + cardi/o + -ia). Use brady- to form a word that means decreased pulse rate: _____

arterioles

20. You learned in Figure 6-1 that arteries branch out to form _____.

capillaries

21. Arterioles carry blood to the smallest blood vessels, the _____, where exchange of oxygen and carbon dioxide occurs.

venules

22. Small vessels that collect blood from the capillaries are _____.

phleb/o, ven/o

23. Veins carry blood back to the heart. Write the two combining forms that mean vein: _____ and _____

phlebitis[79]

24. Use phleb/o to write a word that means inflammation of a vein: _____

vein

25. Thrombo/phleb/itis[80] is inflammation of a _____ associated with a blood clot. Thromb/o is a combining form for thrombus,[81] or blood clot. You should know that some specialists differentiate between a blood clot (occurring outside the body) and a thrombus (occurring internally).

---

[77] tak″e kar′de ah
[78] brad″e kar′de ah
[79] flĕ bi′tis

[80] throm″bo fle bi′tis
[81] throm′bus

vein

26. Ven/ous[82] means pertaining to the veins. Venous thromb/osis[83] is a blood clot in a _____. This can be caused by an injury to the leg or prolonged bed confinement, or it can be a complication of phlebitis.

varicose

27. Varicose[84] veins are swollen and knotted, and occur most often in the legs. They result from defective valves in the veins and sluggish blood flow. Defective valves allow the blood to collect in the veins. A varicose vein is also called a varicosity.[85] Swollen and knotted veins are called _____ veins.

hemorrhoids

28. Hemorrhoids[86] are masses of dilated, varicose veins in the anal[87] canal. Hemorrhoids are often accompanied by pain, itching, and bleeding. A hemorrhoid/ectomy[88] is surgical excision of _____ .

vein

29. Phleb/ectomy[89] is surgical excision of a _____ or of a segment of it.

vein

30. You have already learned that venous thrombosis is the presence of a thrombus (blood clot) in a _____ .

thrombus

31. Thromb/osis is the formation, development, or presence of a _____ .

brain

32. A cerebral thrombosis is formation of a thrombus in a vessel of the _____ .

coronary

33. Remember that coronary arteries supply blood to the heart. Formation of a blood clot in a coronary artery, which then leads to occlusion of the vessel, is called _____ thrombosis. This is a common cause of myocardial infarction.

---

[82] ve′nus
[83] throm bo′sis
[84] var′ĭ kōs
[85] var″ĭ kos′ĭ te

[86] hem′o roidz
[87] a′nal
[88] hem″o roid ek′to me
[89] fle bek′to me

34. An embolism[90] is the sudden blocking of an artery or lymph vessel by foreign material that has been brought to the site of blockage by the circulating blood. The foreign material brought to the vessel is called an embolus.[91]

clot

35. A thrombotic[92] (thromb/o + -tic, pertaining to) embolus is a blood _____ that has broken loose from its place of origin and has been brought to an artery or lymph vessel by the circulating blood.

36. Emboli[93] (plural of embolus) can be bits of tissue, tumor cells, globules of fat, air bubbles, clumps of bacteria, blood clots, or other material. If the embolus is a blood clot, it is called a _____ embolus.

thrombotic

EXERCISE V

Match the combining forms in the left column with their meanings in the right column.

_____ 1. angi/o   A. blood clot
_____ 2. ather/o   B. yellow, fatty plaque
_____ 3. phleb/o   C. vein
_____ 4. thromb/o   D. vessel
_____ 5. vas/o

EXERCISE VI

Using word parts you have learned, write letters in the blanks to complete each sentence.

1. Hardening of the arteries is __ __ __ __ __ __ __sclerosis.
2. Inflammation of the aorta is __ __ __ __itis.
3. Angio__ __ __ __ __ __graphy is roentgenography of the heart and great vessels.
4. Stroke or stroke syndrome is also called a cerebro-__ __ __ __ __ __ __ __ accident.
5. Inflammation of a vein associated with a blood clot is thrombo__ __ __ __ __itis.

[90] em′bo lizm
[91] em′bo lus
[92] throm bot′ik
[93] em′bo lī

6. A disease that involves inflammation of many arteries is called poly — — — — — — — — —.

EXERCISE VII

Match the definitions in the left column with the appropriate terms in the right column (not all selections will be used).

_____ 1. radiography of the vessels

_____ 2. formation of a blood clot in a vessel or cavity of the heart

_____ 3. ballooning out of the wall of a vessel

_____ 4. increased pulse rate

A. aortitis
B. arteritis
C. aneurysm
D. angiography
E. bradycardia
F. tachycardia
G. thrombosis

(Check your answers.)

THE BLOOD

Blood circulates through the heart, arteries, veins, and capillaries and carries oxygen, nourishment, vitamins, antibodies, and other needed substances. It carries away waste matter and carbon dioxide. Approximately half of the blood is composed of cells, and the remainder is a straw-colored fluid, **plasma.** In a **blood transfusion,** blood from the donor is transferred into a blood vessel of the patient, the recipient of the blood. Some blood transfusions require the use of **whole blood,** blood treated with a substance called an **anticoagulant**[94] (anti-, against) to prevent it from clotting. Blood coagulates[95] (clots) if it is not treated with an anticoagulant when removed from the body. In other types of transfusions, only part of the blood is needed. The white cells, red cells, plasma, and blood platelets are blood fractions that can be used in a transfusion. A **transfusion reaction** is any adverse effect that occurs after transfusion. There are many types of reactions, ranging from acute reactions, which are life-threatening, to relatively benign allergic reactions.

Hematology[96] is the study of blood and the blood-forming tissues. The blood-forming tissues are bone marrow and lymphoid[97] tissue (spleen, tonsils, and lymph nodes). Hemat/o means blood, but in the

---

[94] an″tĭ ko ag′u lant
[95] ko ag′u lātz
[96] hem″ah tol′o je
[97] lim′foid

word *hematology,* the definition includes the blood-forming tissues. A **hematoma**[98] (hemat/o + -oma, tumor) is a localized collection of blood, usually clotted, in an organ, tissue, or space, resulting from a break in the wall of a blood vessel. Hematomas can occur almost anywhere in the body and are usually not serious. Bruises are familiar forms of hematomas. Hematomas that occur inside the skull, however, are dangerous. The word *hematoma* is derived from the old meaning of tumor, a swelling, so named because there is a raised area wherever a hematoma occurs.

Blood clots when it is removed from the body; this is called **blood coagulation.**[99] A substance that delays or prevents blood from clotting is an **anticoagulant.** Blood can be treated with an anticoagulant as soon as it is removed from the body, which prevents coagulation. Some patients tend to form clots within blood vessels. Thrombosis, formation of internal blood clots, is a serious condition that can result in death. Special anticoagulant therapy is indicated for such persons to prevent internal clot formation.

You learned earlier that -cyte, erythr/o, and leuk/o mean cell, red, and white, respectively. Two major types of cells (also called corpuscles) are found in the blood, erythro/cytes and leuko/cytes. **Erythrocytes**[100] are red blood cells and appear as biconcave disks that do not normally have a nucleus in circulating blood. Erythrocytes contain **hemoglobin**[101] (hem/o, blood, + globin, a type of protein). Hemoglobin is a red, iron-containing pigment that transports oxygen to the tissues and waste carbon dioxide to the lungs, where it is exchanged for fresh oxygen. **Anemia**[102] (an-, without, + -emia, blood) is a condition in which the number of red blood cells, concentration of hemoglobin, or both are decreased. **Pallor**[103] (paleness) and tachycardia are some typical signs of mild anemia, whereas more serious problems, such as difficulty in breathing, shortness of breath (SOB), headache, fainting, and even congestive heart failure can occur in severe anemia.

There are many types of **leukocytes,**[104] white blood cells, in normal blood. Their major function is body defense, helping to combat infection. Many leukocytes are markedly phagocytic (phag/o, eat, + cyt/o, cell). **Phagocytes**[105] are cells that can ingest and destroy particulate substances such as bacteria, protozoa, cells, and cell debris. **Leukopenia**[106] or **leukocytopenia**[107] (-penia, deficiency) is an abnor-

---

[98] hem'ah to'mah

[99] ko ag"u la'shun

[100] ĕ rith'ro sītz

[101] he'mo glo"bin

[102] ah ne'me ah

[103] pal'or

[104] loo'ko sītz

[105] fag'o sītz

[106] loo"ko pe'ne ah

[107] loo"ko si to pe'ne ah

mal decrease in the total number of white blood cells. **Leukocytosis**[108] is an abnormal increase in the total number of white blood cells. Leukocytosis can be transitory, but it is often associated with a bacterial infection.

Leukemia[109] (-emia, blood) is a progressive, malignant disease of the blood-forming organs. It is characterized by a marked increase in the number of leukocytes and by the presence of immature forms of leukocytes in the blood and bone marrow. Leukemias are classified according to the type of leukocyte in greatest number and according to the severity of the disease (acute or chronic).

Blood platelets are small formed elements in the blood that are important for blood clotting (Fig. 6–2). Blood platelets are also called **thrombocytes**[110] (thromb/o, blood clot, + -cyte, cell), but they are not really cells, only cell fragments. A reduction below normal in the number of blood platelets is called **thrombocytopenia**[111] or **thrombopenia**[112] (-penia, deficiency). This results in a prolonged clotting time.

EXERCISE VIII

Match clues in the left column with the answers in the right column (the choices on the right may be used more than once).

_____ 1. red blood cell
_____ 2. white blood cell
_____ 3. cell responsible for transporting oxygen
_____ 4. red pigment in blood
_____ 5. cell that is often decreased in anemia
_____ 6. major cell type that is increased in leukemia
_____ 7. has an important function in blood clotting

A. blood platelet
B. erythrocyte
C. hemoglobin
D. leukocyte

---

[108] loo″ko si to′sis
[109] loo ke′me ah
[110] throm′bo sītz

[111] throm″bo si″to pe′ne ah
[112] throm″bo pe′ne ah

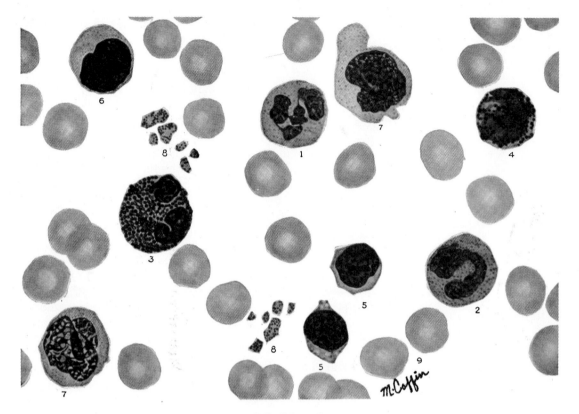

FIGURE 6-2

Types of human blood cells (stained). Shown here are white blood cells, or leukocytes *(1–7)*, platelets *(8)*, and red blood cells, or erythrocytes *(9)*. The white cells (leukocytes) are active in the immune response (defense against disease). The several different types of leukocytes can be identified by the shape of their nucleus and the size and color of the granules in their cytoplasm: segmented neutrophil *(1)*; nonsegmented neutrophil, called a neutrophilic stab *(2)*; eosinophil *(3)*; basophil *(4)*; small lymphocytes *(5)*; large lymphocyte *(6)*; and monocytes *(7)*. The platelets, or thrombocytes *(8)*, are involved in clotting, and the red blood cells, or erythrocytes *(9)*, carry oxygen. (From Custer, R. P. (ed.): *An Atlas of the Blood and Bone Marrow*. 2nd ed. Philadelphia, W. B. Saunders, 1974.)

EXERCISE IX

Use one of the following words or word parts to correctly complete each sentence. (These are shown without hyphens and slashes to make the exercise more challenging.)

an	cyte	graphy	oma
algia	di	immune	osis
ante	emia	ist	penia
anti			vaso

1. A substance that delays or prevents blood from clotting is an
   __ __ __ __coagulant.
2. A localized collection of blood in an organ, tissue, or space of the
   body is a hemat __ __ __.
3. A deficiency of red cells and/or hemoglobin is __ __emia.
4. A cell that ingests particulate substances such as bacteria or dead
   cells is a phago __ __ __ __.
5. A decrease in the number of white blood cells is called leuko-
   __ __ __ __ __.

(Check your answers.)

THE LYMPHATIC SYSTEM

The lymphatic system is also called the **lymphatics.** The primary function of the lymphatic system is to collect fluid that escapes from the blood capillaries and return it to the circulation. As blood circulates, some of the fluid leaves the capillaries to bathe the tissue cells. Thin-walled lymphatic vessels, distributed throughout the body, collect the escaped fluid. If the lymphatics become obstructed, fluid collects in the tissue and swelling results. Swelling that is caused by the obstruction of a lymphatic vessel is called **lymphedema.**[113] Lymph/o either refers to the lymphatics or to the fluid **lymph,** which is the fluid transported by the lymphatic vessels.

The lymph vessels, lymph nodes, lymph, tonsils, thymus, and spleen compose the lymphatic system. Small knots of tissue found at intervals along the course of the lymphatic vessels are called the **lymph nodes.** When cancer is present, the lymphatic system frequently becomes involved in the spread of the disease. If cancer cells wander into a lymphatic vessel, the cells may be trapped by the lymph nodes and begin growing there, or the cells may be carried to sites far from their origin. Cancer occurring within the lymphatic system is called **lymphatic carcinoma.** Usually cancer spreads to the lymphatics from another site rather than originating there. **Lymphoma**[114] (lymph/o, lymphatic, + -oma, tumor) is a general term for cancer originating within the lymphatic system.

Lymphangitis[115] (angi/o, vessel, + -itis, inflammation) is an acute or chronic inflammation of lymphatic vessels, and can be caused by various microorganisms. **Lymphangiography**[116] is roentgenography of the lymphatic vessels and nodes after injection of a radiopaque substance has made them visible on x-ray. **Lymphangio-**

---

[113] lim″fĕ de′mah
[114] lim fo′mah

[115] lim″fan ji′tis
[116] lim fan″je og′rah fe

grams[117] are useful for checking the integrity of the lymphatic system in lymphedema and for investigating tumors.

The lymph nodes were once considered to be glands, so the word part *aden/o* often appears in terms related to the lymph nodes. **Lymphadenitis**[118] is inflammation of the lymph nodes, **lymphadenopathy**[119] (-pathy, disease) refers to any disease of the lymph nodes, and **lymphadenoma**[120] (-oma, swelling) is enlargement of the lymph nodes.

The lymphatic system includes the tonsils and spleen. **Splenomegaly**[121] (splen/o, spleen, + -megaly, enlargement) means enlarged spleen. Hemorrhage can occur if the spleen is ruptured by a crushing injury to the abdomen, and a **splenectomy**[122] (-ectomy, excision), surgical removal of the spleen, would probably be necessary to prevent the patient from bleeding to death.

The **tonsils** are masses of lymphatic tissue located in depressions of the mucous membranes of the pharynx. We usually think of tonsils as the small masses located at the back of the throat, but these are just one type of tonsil, the **palatine tonsils.**[123] The combining form tonsill/o generally refers to the palatine tonsil, as in **tonsillectomy**[124] (excision of the tonsils) or **tonsillitis**[125] (inflammation of the tonsils). **Pharyngeal**[126] **tonsils** are commonly called **adenoids.**[127] An **adenoidectomy**[128] (adenoid/o, adenoid) is often performed at the same time as a tonsillectomy, and is abbreviated T & A. When the component parts of the term *adenoid* are analyzed, they mean resembling a gland (aden/o + -oid). For this reason, pharyngeal tonsils is a more appropriate name for these masses of tissue.

Several new word parts have been introduced in this chapter and appear in the following list. Be sure that you **recognize their meanings.**

ADDITIONAL WORD PARTS AND THEIR MEANINGS

Word Part	Meaning
adenoid/o	adenoids
ather/o	yellow, fatty plaque

---

[117] lim fan′je o gramz
[118] lim fad″ě ni′tis
[119] lim fad ě nop′ah the
[120] lim″fad ě no mah
[121] sple″no meg′ah le
[122] sple nek′to me

[123] pal′ah tīn ton′silz
[124] ton″sĭ lek′to me
[125] ton″sĭ li′tis
[126] fah rin′je al
[127] ad′ě noidz
[128] ad ě noid ek′to me

ADDITIONAL WORD PARTS AND THEIR MEANINGS (Continued)

Word Part	Meaning
ech/o, son/o	sound
-emia, hem/a, hem/o	blood
extra-	outside
home/o	sameness
lymph/o	lymph or lymphatics
lymphat/o	lymphatics
my/o	muscle
pulmon/o	lung
radi/o	radiant energy (this combining form is also used for radius, a bone of the forearm)
splen/o	spleen
thromb /o	thrombus, blood clot

EXERCISE X

Match the meanings in the left column with the medical terms in the right column (not all selections will be used).

_____ 1. swelling caused by obstruction of a lymphatic tissue

_____ 2. general term for cancer originating in the lymphatic system

_____ 3. inflammation of the lymphatic vessels

_____ 4. record produced by x-ray of the lymphatic vessels and nodes

_____ 5. any disease of the lymph nodes

A. lymphadenitis
B. lymphadenoma
C. lymphadenopathy
D. lymphangiogram
E. lymphangiography
F. lymphangitis
G. lymphedema
H. lymphoma
I. lymphosarcoma

(Check your answers.)

Comprehensive Review Exercises

WORK THE FOLLOWING EXERCISES TO TEST YOUR UNDERSTANDING OF THE
MATERIAL IN CHAPTER 6. IT IS BEST TO WORK ALL THE REVIEW EXERCISES
BEFORE CHECKING YOUR ANSWERS.

A. Write the meaning of each underlined word part.

1. cardio<u>pulmon</u>ary _____

2. lymph<u>angi</u>oma _____

3. <u>vas</u>oconstriction _____

4. <u>ather</u>osclerosis _____

5. <u>ven</u>ous _____

6. <u>adenoid</u>ectomy _____

7. <u>son</u>ogram _____

8. <u>hem</u>angioma _____

9. an<u>emia</u> _____

10. <u>myo</u>cardium _____

11. <u>splen</u>omegaly _____

12. <u>hemat</u>ology _____

13. <u>thromb</u>us _____

14. <u>echo</u>cardiography _____

**B. Match the meanings in the left column with the answers in the
right column (the choices on the right may be used more than once).**

_____ 1. cell responsible for transporting oxygen	A. blood platelet
	B. erythrocyte
	C. hemoglobin
_____ 2. cell responsible for transporting carbon dioxide	D. leukocyte
_____ 3. red pigment of blood	
_____ 4. has an important function in coagulation	
_____ 5. cell that functions primarily in body defense	

C. Using words or word parts you have learned, write letters in the blanks to complete each sentence.

1. A soft blowing or rasping heart sound is called a heart __ __ __ __ __ __.

2. Inflammation of many arteries is poly __ __ __ __ __ __ __ __ __.

3. Decreased pulse rate is __ __ __ __ __cardia.

4. Inflammation of a vein associated with a blood clot is thrombo __ __ __ __ __itis.

5. Swelling that results from obstruction of a lymphatic vessel is lymph __ __ __ __ __.

6. Roentgenography of the lymphatic vessels and nodes is lymph __ __ __ __ __graphy.

D. Write the medical term for which each meaning is given.

1. enlarged heart _____

2. elevated blood pressure _____

3. increased pulse rate _____

4. inflammation of the aorta _____

5. hardening of the arteries _____

6. development or formation of a thrombus _____

7. excision of the spleen _____

8. inflammation of the lymphatic vessels _____

E. Circle the correct answer to complete each sentence.

1. Inflammation of the lining of the heart is (endocarditis, polyarteritis, myocarditis, pericarditis).

2. (Cardiovascular, Circulation, Hemangioma, Interstitial) pertains to the heart and blood vessels.

3. Death of part of the heart muscle is (angina pectoris, congestive heart failure, myocardial infarction, myocardial ischemia).

4. A general term that designates primary myocardial disease is (cardiomyopathy, congenital heart defect, heart block, ischemia).

5. A severe cardiac arrhythmia in which contractions are rapid, uncoordinated, and ineffective is (cardiopulmonary resuscitation, catheterization, coronary heart disease, fibrillation).

6. An excessive quantity of fat in the blood is (hyperkalemia, hyperlipemia, hypernatremia, hypertension).

7. The use of ultrasound in diagnosing heart disease is (cardiac catheterization, computed tomography, echocardiography, electrocardiography).
8. Intercellular or interstitial fluid is the same as (intracellular fluid, plasma, serum, tissue fluid).
9. Ballooning out of the wall of a vessel, usually an artery, because of a congenital defect or weakness of the vessel wall, is called (an aneurysm, an embolus, a hemorrhoid, a thrombus).
10. The sudden blocking of an artery or lymph vessel by foreign material that has been brought there by the circulating blood is called (arteritis, embolism, lymphedema, varicosity).
11. A substance that delays or prevents blood from clotting is (an anticoagulant, a coagulation, a phagocyte, a thrombocyte).
12. Cells that can ingest and destroy particulate substances are called (erythrocytes, phagocytes, sickle cells, thrombocytes).
13. The fluid transported by lymphatic vessels is (lymph, lymphoma, plasma, serum).
14. Any disease of the lymph nodes is a (lymphadenitis, lymphadenopathy, lymphadenoma, lymphangiography).

7

The Respiratory System

OBJECTIVES

After completing Chapter 7, you will be able to

1. Match the organs of respiration with their common names, where appropriate.
2. Write the meanings of the word parts pertaining to the respiratory system that are presented in this chapter and choose the correct meaning when presented with several answers.
3. Analyze terms related to the respiratory system, select the appropriate response when presented with several answers, and write the term when presented with its definition.

OUTLINE

RESPIRATION AND ITS FUNCTION
RESPIRATORY STRUCTURES
TERMS PERTAINING TO SURGICAL PROCEDURES
DISEASES, DISORDERS, AND DIAGNOSTIC TERMS
COMPREHENSIVE REVIEW EXERCISES

RESPIRATION AND ITS FUNCTION

Respiration[1] is the combined activity of various processes that supply oxygen to all body cells and remove carbon dioxide. Breathing is **external respiration,** the absorption of oxygen from the air and the removal of carbon dioxide by the lungs. The **respiratory**[2] **system** consists of a series of passages that bring outside air into contact with special structures that lie close to blood capillaries. Oxygen and carbon dioxide are exchanged at the interface between these special structures and the capillaries. This exchange of gases is essential for homeostasis (home/o, sameness, + -stasis, controlling). **Homeostasis**[3] is the state of equilibrium of the internal environment of the body.

Breathing consists of the **inspiration**[4] (in-, in, + spir/o, to breathe) and **expiration**[5] (ex-, out) of air into and out of the lungs. Inspiration is also called **inhalation**[6] whereas expiration is **exhalation.**[7]

Dyspnea[8] is labored or difficult breathing. Dyspnea is derived from dys-, meaning difficult, and -pnea, meaning breathing. **A/pnea**[9] (a-, without) means temporary absence of breathing. Perhaps you have heard of sleep apnea, a condition in which brief absence of breathing is most pronounced while a person is sleeping. **Orthopnea**[10] (orth/o, straight) is a respiratory condition in which there is breathing discomfort in any position except sitting erect or standing.

Normal respiration in an adult consists of 15 to 20 breaths/minute. Abnormally slow breathing is **bradypnea**[11] (brady-, slow). Respiration is considered to be accelerated when it exceeds 25 breaths/minute. This is called **tachypnea**[12] (tachy-, fast), and it may be the result of exercise or physical exertion, but frequently occurs in disease. **Hyperpnea**[13] (hyper-, more than normal) is an increased respiratory rate or breathing that is deeper than normal. Whereas a certain degree of hyperpnea is normal after exercise, it can also result from pain, respiratory or heart disease, or several other conditions.

Spirometry[14] (spir/o, to breathe, + -metry, measurement) is measurement of the amount of air taken into and expelled from the lungs. The largest volume of air that can be exhaled after maximum inspiration is the **vital capacity.** A reduction in vital capacity often indicates a loss of functioning lung tissue. Inability of the lungs to perform their ventilatory function is **acute respiratory failure.** This

---

[1] res″pĭ ra′shun
[2] re spi′rah to″re, res′pĭ rah to″re
[3] ho″me o sta′sis
[4] in″spĭ ra′shun
[5] eks″pĭ ra′shun
[6] in″hah la′shun
[7] eks″hah la′shun

[8] disp′ne ah
[9] ap ne′ah
[10] or″thop ne′ah
[11] brad″e ne′ah
[12] tak″ip ne′ah
[13] hi″perp ne′ah
[14] spi rom′ĕ tre

leads to **hypoxia**[15] (hypo-, less than normal, + ox/o, oxygen) or to **anoxia**[16] (an-, absence). Both terms mean a deficiency of oxygen, which can be caused by respiratory disorders but can also occur under other conditions. Hypoxia can be caused by a lowered oxygen concentration in inspired air at high altitudes or by anemia (decrease in hemoglobin, number of erythrocytes in the blood, or both). When respiratory failure occurs, external support by **artificial respiration** is usually indicated. A **ventilator**[17] is a machine that is used for prolonged artificial ventilation of the lungs.

The meanings of several word parts are given in the preceding paragraphs, but you probably remember many of them from Chapters 2 and 3. Four new word parts are presented in the following list. Be sure to commit their meaning to **memory**.

WORD PARTS PERTAINING TO RESPIRATION

Word Part	Meaning
home/o	sameness
ox/o	oxygen
-pnea	breathing
spir/o	to breathe

EXERCISE I

Match the terms in the right column with their meanings in the left column (not all selections will be used).

_E_ 1. breathing air into the lungs

_C_ 2. labored or difficult breathing

_B_ 3. abnormally slow breathing

_F_ 4. acceleration in the number of breaths per minute

_A_ 5. a deficiency of oxygen

A. anoxia
B. bradypnea
C. dyspnea
D. expiration
E. inspiration
F. tachypnea

[15] hi pok′se ah
[16] ah nok′se ah

[17] ven″tĭ la′tor

EXERCISE II

Using words or word parts you have learned, write letters in the blanks to complete each sentence.

1. A respiratory condition in which breathing is difficult or impossible in any position except sitting erect or standing is
__ __ __ __ __pnea.
2. Equilibrium of the internal environment of the body is
__ __ __ __ __stasis.
3. Measurement of the amount of air taken into and expelled from the lungs is __ __ __ __ __metry.
4. The largest volume of air that can be expelled after maximum inspiration is the __ __ __ __ __ capacity.
5. A machine for prolonged artificial respiration is a __ __ __ __
__ __ __ __ __ __.

(Check your answers with the solutions in the back of the book.)

RESPIRATORY STRUCTURES

The respiratory system consists of the organs involved in the exchange of gases between an organism and the atmosphere. Figure 7–1 shows the major organs of the respiratory system. Label the numbered blanks as you read the information that accompanies the drawing.

The **diaphragm**[18] is a muscular wall that separates the abdomen from the **thoracic**[19] (thorac/o, chest) **cavity.** The diaphragm contracts and relaxes with each inspiration and expiration.

Phrenic[20] means pertaining to the diaphragm, but it sometimes means pertaining to the mind. That is because phren/o means mind or diaphragm. Usually the meaning of phrenic can be determined by how it is used in a sentence.

The chest cavity contains the lungs and many other organs of respiration. Each lung is surrounded by a membrane called the **pleura.**[21] The chest cavity walls are also lined with pleura. The space between the pleura that covers the lungs and the pleura that lines the thoracic cavity is called the **pleural cavity. Pleuritis**[22] (pleur/o means pleura), also called **pleurisy,**[23] is inflammation of the pleura. It can be caused by infection, injury, or tumor, or it can be a complication of certain lung diseases. It is characterized by a sharp pain on inspiration.

---

[18] di'ah fram
[19] tho ras' ik
[20] fren'ik

[21] ploor'ah
[22] ploo ri'tis
[23] ploor'ĭ se

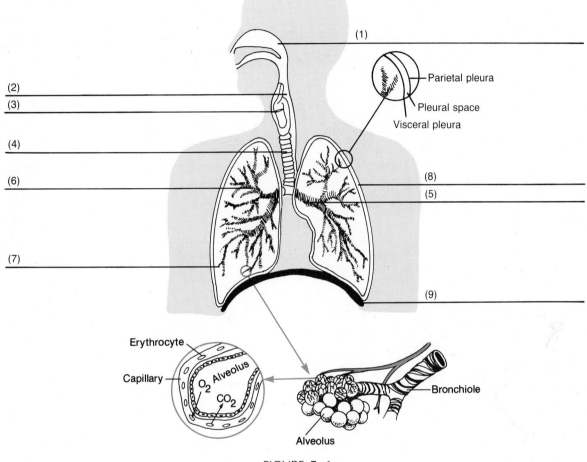

(1)

Parietal pleura

Pleural space

Visceral pleura

(2)

(3)

(4)

(6)   (8)

(5)

(7)

(9)

Erythrocyte

Capillary

O_2 Alveolus

CO_2

Bronchiole

Alveolus

FIGURE 7–1

The organs of respiration. Air first enters the body through the nose and passes through the **nasal cavity** *(1)*. It reaches the **pharynx** *(2)* and passes to the **larynx** *(3)* and the **trachea** *(4)*. The trachea divides into two **bronchi.** Label the bronchus shown *(5)*. Each bronchus divides into smaller tubes called **bronchioles** *(6)*. At the end of each bronchiole are clusters of air sacs called **alveoli** *(7)*. Here oxygen is exchanged for waste carbon dioxide. Each lung is encased in a membrane called the **pleura** *(8)*. Normal quiet breathing is accomplished almost entirely by movement of the **diaphragm** *(9)*. (From Leonard, P.C.: *Building a Medical Vocabulary*. 2nd ed. Philadelphia, W.B. Saunders, 1988).

Commit the following word parts and their meanings to **memory**. After you have studied the list, cover the left column and check to make sure that you know the combining form(s) for each structure before proceeding to the programmed learning section.

COMBINING FORMS THAT PERTAIN TO RESPIRATORY STRUCTURES

Combining Form	Meaning
alveol/o	alveolus[24]
bronch/o, bronchi/o	bronchi[25]
bronchiol/o	bronchiole[26]
laryng/o	larynx[27]
phren/o	diaphragm (this sometimes means mind)
pleur/o	pleura
nas/o, rhin/o	nose
pharyng/o	pharynx[28]
pneum/o, pneumon/o, pulm/o, pulmon/o	lung (pneum/o and pneumon/o sometimes mean air)
thorac/o	chest
trache/o	trachea[29] (windpipe)

PROGRAMMED LEARNING

Remember to cover the answers in the left column. Write answers in the blank spaces and then check each answer by sliding the card down as you work each frame.

---

pneum/o, pneumon/o	1. Four combining forms in the previous list refer to the lungs, but two of the word parts can also mean air. Write the combining forms that mean lung, but in some words can mean air: _____ and _____

---

[24] al ve′o lus
[25] brong′ki
[26] brong′ke ōl

[27] lar′inks
[28] far′inks
[29] tra′ke ah

air	2. Pneum/atic[30] has more than one meaning. It can pertain to respiration or _____, and sometimes even to rarefied or compressed air (as in pneumatic tires).
lungs	3. Pneumo/cardial,[31] however, refers to the _____ and heart. (Decide whether *lung* or *air* is the appropriate response.)
lung	4. Pneumon/ectomy[32] means removal of _____ tissue, and involves removal of all or part of the lung.
pneumectomy[33]	5. Use pneum/o to build another word that means removal of lung tissue: _____
air	6. Thorax[34] means chest. Pneumo/thorax refers to air or gas in the chest cavity, specifically the pleural cavity. Pneumo/hemo/thorax[35] means the presence of _____ and blood in the pleural cavity.
lungs	7. Pneumonia[36] or pneumon/itis[37] means inflammation of the _____. There are many causes of pneumonia, but it is caused primarily by bacteria, viruses, or chemical irritants.
bronchi	8. Broncho/pneumonia[38] is inflammation of the lungs and of the _____.
pneumocentesis[39]	9. Use pneum/o to build a word that means surgical puncture of a lung: _____ (Congratulations if you remembered the suffix that means surgical puncture!)
lungs	10. Pulmon/ary[40] and pulmon/ic[41] both refer to the _____.

[30] nu mat'ik
[31] nu"mo kar'de al
[32] nu"mo nek'to me
[33] nu mek'to me
[34] tho'raks
[35] nu"mo he"mo tho'raks

[36] nu mo'ne ah
[37] nu"mo ni'tis
[38] brong"ko nu mo'ne ah
[39] nu"mo sen te'sis
[40] pul'mo ner"e
[41] pul mon'ik

lungs

11. Pulmonary edema[42] is effusion (escape) of fluid into the air spaces and tissue spaces of the _____ (edema is abnormal accumulation of fluid in the tissue). Although pulmonary edema can have other causes, a major cause is insufficient cardiac activity. Remember that cardi/o means heart, so cardi/ac refers to the heart.

breathing

12. Dyspnea on exertion is one of the earliest symptoms of pulmonary edema. As the condition becomes more advanced, the patient can become ortho/pneic,[43] which means that _____ is difficult except when the patient is sitting erect or standing.

pulmonary

13. Pulmonary arteries carry blood from the heart to the lungs so carbon dioxide can be exchanged for oxygen. A pulmonary embolus[44] is an obstruction of the _____ artery or one of its branches.

pulmonary

14. Embolism[45] is the sudden blocking of an artery by foreign material that has been brought to its site of blockage by the circulating blood. An embolus is often a blood clot, called a thrombus.[46] The pulmonary artery is obstructed in _____ embolism.

lobe

15. Each lung is divided into lobes. A lob/ectomy[47] (lob/o, lobe) is excision of a _____. Because other organs such as the liver and brain also have lobes, one has to say pulmonary lobectomy unless it is clear that the lobectomy refers to the lung.

16. Air usually first enters the respiratory passageway through the nose, which refers to the external nose as well as the nasal cavity. Write the two combining forms that mean nose: _____ and _____

nas/o
rhin/o

17. The nares,[48] or nostrils, are the external openings of the nose. These openings lead into two nasal cavities separated by the

---

[42] ĕ de'mah
[43] or"thop ne'ik
[44] em'bo lus
[45] em'bo lizm

[46] throm'bus
[47] lo bek'to me
[48] na'rēz

nasal	nasal septum. The partition between the two nasal cavities is the _____ septum.
nose	18. The para/nasal[49] (para-, near or beside) sinuses open into the nasal cavities. The term *sinus* has several meanings, including canal, passage, and cavity within a bone. The paranasal sinuses are cavities within the bones of the face. Fluids from the paranasal sinuses are discharged into the _____.
sinus	19. Sinus/itis[50] is inflammation of a _____, especially of a paranasal sinus.
rhin/o	20. You learned that, in addition to nas/o, another combining form that means nose is _____.
rhinitis[51]	21. Use rhin/o to build a term that means inflammation of the nasal membrane: _____.
nose	22. Rhino/rrhea[52] is a watery discharge from the _____.
pharynx	23. Air from the nose passes to the pharynx, commonly called the throat. Pharyng/eal[53] pertains to the _____.
nose **pharynx**	24. Naso/pharyng/eal[54] pertains to the _____ and _____.
inflammation	25. Pharyng/itis[55] is _____ of the pharynx.
pharynx	26. The eustachian[56] or auditory[57] tube extends from the middle ear to the pharynx. It is sometimes called the oto/pharyngeal[58] tube, meaning a tube that communicates with the ear and _____.

[49] par″ah na′sal
[50] si nŭ si′tis
[51] ri ni′tis
[52] ri″no re′ah
[53] fah rin′je al

[54] na″zo fah rin′je al
[55] far″in ji′tis
[56] u sta′ke an
[57] aw′dĭ to″re
[58] o″to fah rin′je al

larynx

27. The lower part of the pharynx is also called the laryngophar-ynx,[59] because it is here that the pharynx divides into the larynx and the esophagus. Air passes to the _____ and food passes to the esophagus.

laryngitis[60]

28. Inflammation of the larynx is _____. This condition can be caused not only by infectious microorganisms, but also by overuse of the voice, allergies, or irritants.

aphonia

29. Laryngitis can result in absence of voice. A/phon/ia[61] means absence of voice. Sounds cannot be produced from the larynx (phon/o means voice). Laryngitis can cause absence of voice, which is called _____.

voice

30. Dys/phonia[62] means difficulty in speaking or a weak _____. Dysphonia is the same as hoarseness, and may precede aphonia.

speech

31. A/phasia[63] is the inability to communicate through speech, writing, or signs. It is caused by improper functioning of the brain. The combining form phas/o means speech. The term a/phas/ia describes only one aspect of the condition, which is the absence of _____.

aphasia

32. An a/phasic individual is one affected by _____. Remember that in aphasia the problem does not arise in the larynx, but in the brain.

speech

33. Dys/phasia[64] is a speech impairment resulting from a brain lesion. There is a lack of coordination and an inability to arrange words in their proper order. In dys/phasia there is difficulty in _____.

34. Be sure that you know the difference between a/phasia and a/phonia. Both can produce an absence of speech sound. Aphasia

---

[59] lah ring″go far′inks
[60] lar″in ji′tis
[61] a fo′ne ah

[62] dis fo′ne ah
[63] ah fa′ze ah
[64] dis fa′ze ah

aphonia

. . . .

pain

. . . .

glottis

. . . .

trachea

. . . .

inside (or interior)

. . . .

incision

. . . .

tracheostomy[71]

. . . .

is caused by a brain dysfunction, however, and in aphonia the problem involves more of an absence of vocal sounds. In laryngitis, for example, which is more likely to occur, aphasia or aphonia? _____

---

35. Laryngitis can cause only minor discomfort, or the condition can become painful. Laryng/algia[65] is _____ of the larynx.

---

36. The larynx is commonly called the voice box. The vocal apparatus of the larynx is the glottis,[66] which consists of the vocal cords (or folds) and the opening between them. Muscles open and close the glottis during breathing and also regulate the vocal cords during the production of sound. The lidlike structure that covers the larynx during the swallowing of food is called the epiglottis[67] (epi-, above). The epi/glottis lies above the _____.

---

37. Air passes from the larynx to the trachea, or windpipe. Trache/al[68] pertains to the _____.

---

38. Endo/tracheal[69] pertains to the _____ of the trachea. Endotracheal intubation is a procedure in which a tube is placed into the trachea through the mouth or nose, pharynx, and larynx to establish an airway.

---

39. Tracheo/tomy[70] is an _____ of the trachea through the skin and muscles of the neck overlying the trachea.

---

40. Knowing that one definition of *stoma* is an artificially created opening, add a suffix to trache/o to form a new term that means forming an artificial opening in the trachea: _____ (this opening can be temporary or permanent).

---

[65] lar″in gal′je ah
[66] glot′tis
[67] ep″ĭ glot′is
[68] tra′ke al
[69] en″do tra′ke al
[70] tra″ke ot′o me
[71] tra″ke os′to me

bronchitis[72]

41. The trachea divides into two bronchi, one leading to each lung. Use bronch/o to write a word that means inflammation of the mucous membrane of the bronchi: _____

sputum

42. Mucous membranes secrete mucus. Inflammation of the mucous membranes in bronchitis usually leads to the production of sputum, which can be expelled by coughing or clearing the throat. Material raised from inflamed mucous membranes of the respiratory tract and expelled by coughing is called _____.

against

43. Anti/tussives[73] are often used to treat coughs caused by inflammation of the respiratory tract. Anti/tussives are agents that act _____ a cough. In other words, antitussives are used to prevent or relieve a cough. Tussive pertains to a cough. Perhaps you already know that the medical name of whooping cough is pertussis.

bronchi

44. The _____ are examined in a broncho/scopic[74] examination.

pertaining

trachea, bronchi

45. Bronchi/al[75] is an adjective that means _____ to the bronchi. Tracheo/bronchial[76] pertains both to the _____ and the _____.

bronchoscopy[77]

46. Add a suffix to bronch/o to write a word that means a bronchoscopic examination using a bronchoscope: _____

bronchi

47. A broncho/dilator[78] is an agent that causes dilation of the _____. Bronchodilators are used in respiratory conditions that constrict the air passages, such as the allergic reaction that occurs in asthma.[79] These medications expand the bronchi and other air passages.

---

[72] brong ki′tis
[73] an″tĭ tus′ivz
[74] brong″ko skop′ic
[75] brong′ke al

[76] tra″ke o brong′ke al
[77] brong kos′ko pe
[78] brong″ko di la′tor
[79] az′mah

bronchi
little

48. Translated literally, bronchi/oles means little _____.
    You see that -ole means _____. Bronchioles are
    subdivisions of the bronchi.

alveoli

49. At the end of the bronchioles are tiny air sacs called alveoli.
    Alveol/ar[80] pertains to the _____.

alveoli

50. In certain diseases, such as emphysema,[81] destructive changes
    occur in the alveolar walls. These interfere with the exchange
    of oxygen and carbon dioxide. This gas exchange takes place
    by diffusion across the walls of blood capillaries and the
    _____.

EXERCISE III

Match the terms in the right column with their common names in
the left column.

_____ 1. air sacs   A. alveoli
_____ 2. windpipe   B. larynx
_____ 3. voice box   C. pharynx
_____ 4. throat   D. thorax
_____ 5. chest   E. trachea

EXERCISE IV

Write the meaning of each underlined word part in the blank spaces.

1. a<u>phon</u>ia _____
2. <u>bronchoscopy</u> _____
3. endo<u>trache</u>al _____
4. <u>laryng</u>algia _____
5. para<u>nas</u>al _____
6. <u>pharyng</u>eal _____
7. <u>pneumo</u>cardial _____
8. <u>pneumo</u>thorax _____
9. <u>pneumon</u>ectomy _____
10. <u>rhin</u>itis _____

[80] al ve′o lar   [81] em″fĭ se′mah

EXERCISE V

Write letters in the blanks to complete each sentence.

1. Another name for pneumonia is pneumon __ __ __ __.

2. Inflammation of the lungs and the bronchi is
__ __ __ __ __ __ __pneumonia.

3. Excision of a lobe of the lungs is pulmonary
lob__ __ __ __ __ __.

4. Inability of communication through speech, writing, or signs because of a brain dysfunction is a __ __ __ __ __ __.

5. Subdivisions of the bronchi are called bronchi __ __ __s.

(Check your answers.)

TERMS PERTAINING TO SURGICAL PROCEDURES

bronchoscopy (-scopy, viewing): examination of the bronchi through a bronchoscope, an instrument designed to pass through the trachea to allow visual inspection of the tracheobronchial tree

laryngoscopy[82]: examination of the interior of the larynx

lung biopsy: removal of small pieces of lung tissue for the purpose of diagnosis. An **open lung biopsy** is one in which a segment of the lung is removed after the surgeon has incised the chest. A **percutaneous**[83] (per-, through, + cutane/o, skin) **biopsy** is one in which tissue is obtained by puncturing the suspected lesion through the skin.

rhinoplasty[84] (rhin/o, nose, + -plasty, surgical repair): plastic surgery of the nose (usually performed for cosmetic reasons, but it might also be necessary to provide a free passageway for respiration)

thoracocentesis[85] (thorac/o, chest, + -centesis, surgical puncture): surgical puncture of the chest cavity to remove fluid (also called thoracentesis or thoracic paracentesis[86])

tracheostomy (trache/o, windpipe, + -stomy, artificial opening): operation of cutting into the trachea through the neck (usually performed for insertion of a tube to relieve tracheal obstruction)

tracheotomy (-tomy, incision): incision of the trachea through the skin and muscles of the neck overlying the trachea

DISEASES, DISORDERS, AND DIAGNOSTIC TERMS

asthma: paroxysmal dyspnea accompanied by wheezing caused by a spasm of the bronchial tubes or by swelling of their mucous membranes. A **wheeze** is a whistling sound made during respiration. **Paroxysmal**[87] means occurring in sudden, periodic attacks or recurrence of symptoms.

atelectasis[88] (atel/o, imperfect, + -ectasis, stretching): a condition in which the lungs of a fetus remain unexpanded at birth, or a collapsed

---

[82] lar″ing gos′ko pe
[83] per″ku ta′ne us
[84] ri′no plas′te
[85] tho″rah ko sen te′sis

[86] par″ah sen te′sis
[87] par″ok siz′mal
[88] at″e lek′tah sis

or airless condition of the lung, usually caused by injury

bronchiectasis[89] (bronchi/o + -ectasis): chronic dilation of a bronchus or bronchi, accompanied by a secondary infection that usually involves the lower part of the lung

bronchography[90] (-graphy, recording): radiography of the bronchi after a radiopaque substance has been injected into them. Radiopaque means not permitting the passage of radiant energy. The record of the bronchi and lungs produced by bronchography is a bronchogram.

COPD: chronic obstructive pulmonary disease, a disease process that decreases the ability of the lungs to perform their ventilatory function. This process can result from chronic bronchitis, emphysema, chronic asthma, and chronic bronchiolitis. COPD is also called chronic obstructive lung disease, or COLD.

emphysema: a chronic pulmonary disease characterized by an increase in the size of alveoli and by destructive changes in their walls, resulting in difficulty in breathing

influenza[91]: an acute, contagious, respiratory infection characterized by sudden onset, chills, headache, fever, and muscular discomfort; it is caused by several different types of viruses

pneumoconiosis[92] (pneum/o, lung, + coni/o, dust): a respiratory condition caused by inhalation of dust particles, more frequently seen in occupations such as mining or stonecutting

RDS: respiratory distress syndrome, a condition that causes many infant deaths each year. Clinical signs, including delayed onset of breathing, are usually present at birth. RDS was formerly known as hyaline membrane disease.

silicosis[93] (silic/o, silica): a form of pneumoconiosis resulting from inhalation of the dust of stone, sand, or flint that contains silica (quartz is a familiar form of silica in its pure state, but silica is present in many materials, particularly glass)

tuberculosis[94] (TB): an infectious disease caused by the bacteria *Mycobacterium tuberculosis*. It is often chronic in nature and commonly affects the lungs, although it can occur elsewhere in the body. The disease is named for the tubercules — small, round nodules — that are produced in the lungs by the bacteria.

Before working the exercises, **review** the list of additional word parts that have been introduced in this chapter.

ADDITIONAL WORD PARTS

Word Part	Meaning
atel/o	imperfect
coni/o	dust
lob/o	lobe
-ole	little
silic/o	silica

[89] brong ke ek'tah sis
[90] brong kog'rah fe
[91] in"flu en'zah
[92] nu"mo ko"ne o'sis
[93] sil"ĭ ko'sis
[94] too ber"ku lo'sis

EXERCISE VI   *Match the medical terms in the right column with their meanings in the left column (not all selections will be used).*

_____ 1. plastic surgery of the nose

_____ 2. surgical puncture of the chest cavity to remove fluid

_____ 3. incision of the windpipe through the neck

_____ 4. x-ray of the bronchi after injection of radiopaque material

_____ 5. visual inspection of the tracheobronchial tree

A. wheeze
B. bronchography
C. bronchoscopy
D. rhinoplasty
E. thoracentesis
F. tracheotomy

EXERCISE VII   *Match the medical terms in the right column with their meanings in the left column (not all selections will be used).*

_____ 1. collapsed condition of the lung

_____ 2. also called chronic obstructive lung disease

_____ 3. chronic disease characterized by increased size of alveoli and destructive changes

_____ 4. condition characterized by dyspnea and wheezing

_____ 5. respiratory condition caused by inhalation of dust particles

A. asthma
B. atelectasis
C. bronchiectasis
D. COPD
E. emphysema
F. influenza
G. pneumoconiosis

(Check your answers.)

Comprehensive Review Exercises

WORK THE FOLLOWING EXERCISES TO TEST YOUR UNDERSTANDING OF THE
MATERIAL IN CHAPTER 7. IT IS BEST TO DO ALL THE REVIEW EXERCISES BEFORE
CHECKING YOUR ANSWERS.

**A. Match the underlined word parts in the left column with their
meanings in the right column (not all selections will be used).**

_____ 1. <u>naso</u>pharyngeal	A. diaphragm
_____ 2. <u>phren</u>ic	B. dust
_____ 3. <u>atel</u>ectasis	C. imperfect
_____ 4. pneumo<u>coni</u>osis	D. little
_____ 5. bronchi<u>ole</u>	E. lung
_____ 6. <u>silic</u>osis	F. nose
	G. silica
	H. speech
	I. throat
	J. voice

B. Write the correct answer in each blank space.

1. The largest volume of air that can be expelled after maximum
   inspiration is _____ capacity.

2. The muscular wall that separates the abdomen from the thoracic
   cavity is the _____.

3. Each lung is surrounded by a membrane called the
   _____.

4. Pneumocardial pertains to the _____ and
   _____.

5. Inflammation of the lungs is called pneumonia, or
   _____.

6. Effusion of fluid into the air spaces and tissue spaces of the lungs
   is called _____ edema.

7. The lidlike structure that covers the larynx during the swallowing of food is called the _____.

8. A respiratory condition characterized by paroxysmal dyspnea
   and wheezing is _____.

9. A chronic disease characterized by increased size of the alveoli
   and destructive changes of their walls is _____.

10. A procedure in which a tube is placed into the trachea through the mouth or nose, pharynx, and larynx to establish an airway is _____ intubation.

C. Circle the correct answer to complete each sentence.

1. Labored or difficult breathing is (bradypnea, dyspnea, hyperpnea, tachypnea).

2. Which of the following is a machine for prolonged artificial respiration? (expirator, ventilator, spirometer, thoracometer)

3. (Pneumatic, pneumohemothorax, pneumonectomy, pneumothorax) is removal of lung tissue.

4. The sudden blocking of an artery by foreign material is called (edema, embolism, lobectomy, pleurisy).

5. Rhinitis is inflammation of the (chest, nose, throat, voice box).

6. Pulmonary refers to the (chest, diaphragm, heart, lungs).

7. Pharyngitis is inflammation of the (chest, nose, throat, voice box).

8. Chronic laryngitis is most likely to cause which of the following? (aphasia, aphonia, olfaction, rales)

9. Material raised from inflamed membranes of the respiratory tract is (emphysema, saliva, sputum, wheeze).

10. An agent used to prevent or relieve a cough is a(n) (antitussive, bronchodilator, epiglottis, rhinorrhea).

11. A disease process that decreases the ability of the lungs to perform their ventilatory function, and that can result from several other chronic disorders of the respiratory organs, is (COPD, hyaline membrane disease, RDS, TB).

12. A term that means pertaining to the windpipe and the bronchi is (bronchiectasis, laryngobronchial, pharyngobronchial, tracheobronchial).

D. Write the medical term for which each meaning is given:

1. respiratory condition in which there is discomfort in breathing in any position except sitting erect or standing _____

2. inflammation of the pleura _____ or _____

3. pertaining to the air sacs of the lung _____

4. radiography of the bronchi after injection of a radiopaque substance _____

5. inflammation of a sinus, especially a paranasal sinus
   _____

6. examination of the interior of the larynx _____

7. plastic surgery of the nose _____

8. chronic dilation of the bronchi _____

8

The Digestive System

OBJECTIVES

> **After completing Chapter 8, you will be able to**
>
> 1. Recognize the meaning and use word parts presented in this chapter that relate to the digestive system.
> 2. Choose the correct definitions for terms and write the appropriate terms when presented with their definition.
> 3. Analyze selected terms related to diagnosis, surgery, and diseases or disorders of the digestive system.

OUTLINE

FUNCTION OF THE DIGESTIVE SYSTEM

STRUCTURES OF THE DIGESTIVE SYSTEM

ACCESSORY ORGANS OF DIGESTION

TERMS PERTAINING TO SURGICAL PROCEDURES

DISEASES, DISORDERS, AND DIAGNOSTIC TERMS

    The mouth

    The esophagus

    The stomach

    The intestines

    The gallbladder

    The liver

    The pancreas

COMPREHENSIVE REVIEW EXERCISES

FUNCTION OF THE DIGESTIVE SYSTEM

Digestion is the process by which food is broken down mechanically and chemically as it is moved along the digestive tract. The digestive system provides nutrition for growth, repair, and maintenance of the body. Lack of proper food or improper absorption and distribution leads to **malnutrition**[1] (mal-, bad). **Anorexia** (an-, without, + -orexia, appetite) is loss of appetite for food. **Anorexia nervosa**[2] is a type of anorexia that cannot be related to a particular disease process, but is believed to be caused by emotional illness. It is a subconscious self-imposed starvation whereby the individual is excessively afraid of

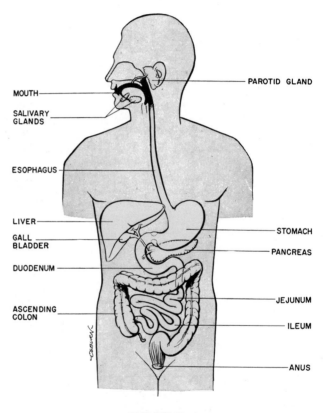

FIGURE 8–1

The digestive system. (From Guyton, A. C.: *Textbook of Medical Physiology.* 6th ed. Philadelphia, W. B. Saunders, 1981.)

---

[1] mal"nu trish'un   [2] an"o rek'se ah ner vo'sah

being obese or overweight. **Hyperemesis**[3] (hyper-, excessive, + -emesis, vomiting) and diarrhea[4] (dia-, through, + -rrhea, discharge) can also interfere with proper nutrition. In addition, either of these conditions can lead to **dehydration**[5] (de-, remove, + hydr/o, water). Dehydration occurs when the output of body fluid exceeds fluid intake. Sufficient water and proper nutrition are essential for body maintenance. **Alimentation**[6] is the process of providing nutrition for the body. For this reason, the digestive tract is also called the **alimentary**[7] **canal** or tract.

STRUCTURES OF THE DIGESTIVE SYSTEM

The digestive system is traditionally divided into the alimentary canal and several organs that are considered accessory organs, because they produce substances needed for proper digestion and absorption of nutrients. The alimentary tract is basically a long, muscular tube that begins at the mouth and ends at the anus. The major organs of digestion are shown in Figure 8–1.

Become familiar with the names of the digestive organs and recognize the parts that make up the small and large intestines. Commit the meaning of the following word parts to **memory.**

WORD PARTS PERTAINING TO DIGESTIVE ORGANS

Word Part	Meaning	
cheil/o	lips	⎫
dent/i, dent/o, odont/o	teeth	
gingiv/o	gums	⎬ mouth and teeth
gloss/o, lingu/o	tongue	
or/o, stomat/o	mouth	⎭
esophag/o	esophagus[8]	
gastr/o	stomach	
intestin/o, enter/o	intestines (enter/o sometimes refers only to the small intestine)	

---

[3] hi″per em′ĕ sis
[4] di″ah re′ah
[5] de hi″dra′shun
[6] al″ĕ men ta′shun
[7] al″ĕ men′tar e
[8] ĕ sof′ah gus

WORD PARTS PERTAINING TO DIGESTIVE ORGANS
(Continued)

Word Part	Meaning	
duoden/o	duodenum[9]	} divisions of the small intestine
jejun/o	jejunum[10]	
ile/o	ileum[11]	
col/o	colon[12] or large intestine*	
append/o, apendic/o	appendix	
cec/o	cecum[13]	} large intestine
proct/o	anus[14] or rectum[15]	
rect/o	rectum	
an/o	anus	

* The colon comprises most of the large intestine. Therefore, *colon* is sometimes used inaccurately as a synonym for the entire large intestine. In words containing col/o, the distinction between the colon or large intestine is usually not significant.

PROGRAMMED LEARNING

Practice using the word parts you have just learned by working the following programmed study. Remember to cover the answers in the left column, and then check each answer after you write it in the blank space.

or/o **stomat/o**	1. The mouth or oral cavity is the beginning of the digestive tract. Write the two word parts that mean mouth: _____ and _____
mouth	2. Stomat/itis[16] is inflammation of the _____.
mouth	3. An oral surgeon is one who specializes in surgery of the _____.

[9] du"o de'num, du od'ĕ num   [13] se'kum
[10] jĕ joo'num   [14] a'nus
[11] il'e um   [15] rek'tum
[12] ko'lon   [16] sto mah ti'tis

gum	4. Gingiva[17] is another name for the gum, the mucous membrane that provides support for the teeth. Gingiv/al[18] pertains to the _____.
gloss/o, lingu/o **glossal,[19] lingual[20]**	5. You have learned that combining forms for tongue are _____ and _____. Use gingival as a model to write two words, both meaning pertaining to the tongue: _____ and _____
under	6. Hypogossal[21] means _____ the tongue.
hypoglossal	7. Certain medications are placed under the tongue, where the medicine dissolves. Write this word that means beneath or under the tongue: _____
teeth	8. The combining forms denti/, dent/o, and odont/o all mean _____.
dental	9. Combine one of the word parts listed in the previous frame with -al to form a commonly used word that means pertaining to the teeth: _____
mouth **teeth**	10. Dentists care for the teeth and associated structures of the oral cavity. Or/al[22] pertains to the _____. There are many dental specialties and most use the word part *odont/o* in forming their names. Ped/odont/ics[23] deals with the _____ and mouth conditions of children.
orthodontist[25]	11. Orth/odont/ics[24] is the branch of dentistry concerned with tooth alignment and associated facial problems. The combining form orth/o means straight or straighten. If someone wished to have his teeth straightened, he would see a specialist in orthodontics, an _____.

[17] jin'jĭ vah, jin ji'vah
[18] jin"jĭ val, jin ji'val
[19] glos'al
[20] ling'gwal
[21] hi"po glos'al

[22] o'ral
[23] pe do don'tiks
[24] or"tho don'tiks
[25] or"tho don'tist

around

12. The tissue that invests and supports the teeth is called perio-dontium.[26] You learned in Chapter 3 that peri- means

_____.

periodontal[27]

13. Use -al to form a word that means pertaining to the peri/odont/ium: _____

periodontium

14. Periodontics[28] is the branch of dentistry that deals with the study and treatment of the _____.

esophagus

15. Food that is swallowed passes from the mouth to the pharynx[29] and then to a long tube called the _____.

esophagus

16. Esophag/eal[30] is an adjective that means pertaining to the _____. (Sometimes the suffix -eal is used instead of -al to form medical terms. Both suffixes mean pertaining to.)

gastr/o

17. The esophagus carries food to the stomach. Write the combining form that means stomach: _____

stomach

18. Gastr/ic[31] means pertaining to the _____.

interior

19. Endogastric[32] means pertaining to the _____ of the stomach.

stomach

20. Washing out of the stomach is called gastric lavage.[33] Lavage means irrigation or washing out of an organ, such as the stomach or bowel. Gastric lavage specifically refers to washing out of the _____. This procedure might be performed to re-move poisonous material or to clean the stomach before gastric surgery.

---

[26] per″e o don′she um
[27] per″e o don′tal
[28] per″e o don′tiks
[29] far′inks

[30] ĕ sof″ah je′al, ĕ so fa′je al
[31] gas′trik
[32] en″do gas′trik
[33] lah vahzh′

pain	21. Gastr/algia[34] and gastro/dynia[35] both mean _____ of the stomach.
intestines	22. Intestin/al[36] pertains to the _____ .
stomach	23. Gastro/intestinal[37] means pertaining to the _____ and the intestines.
duodenum, jejunum ileum	24. The first initials of the three parts of the small intestine are given. They are the d _____ , j _____ , and i _____ .
duodenum	25. Duoden/al[38] pertains to the _____ .
gastroenterologist[40]	26. Gastro/entero/logy[39] is the study of the stomach, intestines, and associated structures. Write the term for a physician who specializes in gastroenterology: _____
liver	27. Bile is a digestive juice produced by the liver. It stimulates movement of food along the alimentary canal and facilitates the digestion of fats. Bile is produced by the _____ .
bile	28. The combining form bil/i means bile. Bili/ary[41] pertains to _____ .
mucus	29. Another factor that facilitates movement of food is the secretion of mucus by the inner lining of the digestive tract. This slimy material is produced by all mucous membranes. Remember that muc/o means _____ .

[34] gas tral'je ah
[35] gas"tro din'e ah
[36] in tes'tĭ nal
[37] gas"tro in tes'tĭ nal
[38] du"o de'nal
[39] gas"tro en"ter ol'o je
[40] gas"tro en"ter ol'o jist
[41] bil'e ar e

ileum cecum	30. The first part of the large intestine is a blind pouch only a few inches long called the cecum. The ileo/cecal[42] valve is a group of muscles that are located between the _____ and the _____.
sigmoid	31. The colon makes up the major portion of the large intestine. The colon is referred to as the ascending, transverse, descending, and sigmoid[43] colon. The latter part of the colon is S-shaped. Hence, it is called the sigmoid colon. Sigmoido/scopy[44] is examination of the _____ colon using an instrument for illumination.
col/o	32. The colon makes up most of the large intestine. Thus, when speaking of the colon, one is often referring to the large intestine in general. The combining form that means colon or large intestine is _____.
rectum	33. The lower part of the large intestine, the rectum, ends in a narrow anal canal, which opens to the exterior at the anus. Rect/al pertains to the _____.
anus	34. Anal[45] pertains to the _____.
anus, rectum	35. The combining form proct/o refers to the anus or the rectum. A procto/logist is a physician who specializes in diseases of the _____ and _____, as well as disorders of the colon.

EXERCISE I

Match the combining forms in the left column with their meanings in the right column (the choices on the right may be used more than once).

_____ 1. cheil/o   A. anus or rectum
_____ 2. col/o   B. gum
_____ 3. dent/o   C. intestines (in general)
                          (This exercise continues on next page.)

---

[42] il″e o se′kal
[43] sig′moid
[44] sig″moi dos′ko pe
[45] a′nal

_____ 4. enter/o   D. large intestine
_____ 5. gastr/o   E. lips
_____ 6. gingiv/o   F. mouth
_____ 7. gloss/o   G. stomach
_____ 8. lingu/o   H. teeth
_____ 9. odont/o   I. tongue
_____ 10. or/o
_____ 11. proct/o
_____ 12. stomat/o

(Check your answers with the solutions in the back of the book.)

ACCESSORY ORGANS OF DIGESTION

The accessory organs of digestion produce substances that are needed for proper digestion and absorption of nutrients. The **liver, gallbladder, pancreas,** and **salivary glands** are **accessory organs** to the digestive system.

The liver is the largest organ in the body. It performs so many vital functions that we cannot live without it. The liver produces **bile,** which is used in the small intestine for the absorption of fats. In certain liver diseases, or if the flow of bile is obstructed, a condition called jaundice can result. **Jaundice**[46] is characterized by yellowness of the skin, whites of the eyes, mucous membranes, and body fluids as a result of deposition of bile pigment.

Bile is transported to the gallbladder for storage. Gallstones sometimes form within the gallbladder and can be lodged there for years without causing problems. If the gallbladder becomes inflamed or swollen, it might become necessary to remove it. If a stone escapes from the gallbladder and obstructs a bile duct, the flow of bile is interrupted. Removal of the gallbladder might also be necessary in these situations.

The pancreas is a small organ with two important functions. It produces pancreatic juice, which is important in the digestion of food. The pancreas also produces **insulin,**[47] a hormone that regulates the blood sugar level. Diminished secretion of insulin results in the condition called **diabetes mellitus.**[48] This disorder leads to **hyperglycemia**[49] (hyper-, increased, + glyc/o, sugar, + -emia, blood), an increased glucose level in the blood. The output of urine is also greatly increased (**polyuria**[50]) in this disorder, and the urine sometimes con-

---

[46] jawn'dis

[47] in'su lin

[48] di"ah be'tez mel'it us

[49] hi"per gli se'me ah

[50] pol"e u're ah

tains glucose (**glycosuria**[51]). (Poly/ur/ia is derived from poly-, many, + ur/o, urine + -ia, condition. Glycos/uria is derived from glycos/o, sugar, + ur/o + -ia.) Another dysfunction of the pancreas is one in which it produces too much insulin and causes **hypoglyce-mia**.[52] In hypoglycemia there is less than the normal amount of sugar in the blood. Remember that hypo- means less than normal.

The salivary[53] glands are located in the oral cavity. **Saliva** is produced by these glands. Saliva contains **amylase**[54] (amyl/o, starch, + -ase, enzyme). Amylase is the enzyme responsible for the breakdown of starch. Because amylase is contained in saliva, starch digestion begins in the mouth.

Commit the meanings of the following word parts to **memory**.

WORD PARTS PERTAINING TO THE ACCESSORY ORGANS OF DIGESTION

Word Part	Meaning
cholecyst/o	gallbladder
hepat/o	liver
pancreat/o	pancreas
sial/o	salivary gland

ADDITIONAL WORD PARTS RELATED TO THE DIGESTIVE SYSTEM

Word Part	Meaning
bil/i, chol/e	bile
muc/o	mucus
-orexia	appetite
-pepsia	digestion
periton/o	peritoneum[55]

---

[51] gli″ko su′re ah
[52] hi″po gli se′me ah
[53] sal′ĭ ver e

[54] am′ĭ lās
[55] per″ĭ to ne′um

EXERCISE II

The first letter of each word part is given after its meaning. Use this clue to write the word part indicated for each of the following:

Meaning	First Letter	Combining Forms
1. pancreas	p	_____
2. liver	h	_____
3. peritoneum	p	_____
4. gallbladder	c	_____
5. salivary gland	s	_____
6. bile	b or c	_____
		_____

Suffixes

7. digestion	p	_____
8. appetite	o	_____

PROGRAMMED LEARNING

Work the following programmed study. Remember to cover the answers in the left column with a folded paper, and then check each answer after you have written it.

appendix	1. The vermiform (worm-shaped) appendix is attached to the cecum. The combining form appendic/o means _____.
appendix	2. Appendicitis[56] is inflammation of the vermiform _____. It is characterized by abdominal pain followed by nausea and vomiting.
appendectomy[57]	3. Inflammation of the appendix can result in the need for its removal. The term that means removal or excision of the appendix is _____. Sometimes the appendix is removed when another surgery is being performed. This is known as an *incidental appendectomy*.

---

[56] ah pen″dĭ si′tis   [57] ap″en dek′to me

hepatitis[58]

4. Other abdominal organs can also become inflamed. Use the combining form you have just learned for liver to write a word that means inflammation of the liver: _____

hepatomegaly[59]

5. When the liver becomes inflamed, it is not unusual for it also to become enlarged. Use a suffix you learned in Chapter 3 to write a word that means enlargement of the liver: _____

liver

6. Cirrhosis[60] is a chronic liver disease characterized by marked degeneration of liver cells. It might be more difficult for you to remember the meaning of cirrhosis, because it does not use a familiar word part. The combining form cirrh/o is derived from a Greek word meaning orange-yellow, but you need to remember that cirrh/osis is a chronic disease of the _____ .

cirrhosis

7. There are other causes of cirrhosis, but a common cause is alcohol abuse. The term for chronic liver disease characterized by marked degeneration of liver cells is _____ .

liver

8. Hepato/toxic[61] means toxic, or destructive, to the _____. Hepatotoxic drugs can damage the liver.

gallbladder

9. Bile is produced by the liver, but stored in the _____. (*Gall* is another term for bile — hence, the use of the term *gallbladder*.)

chol
vessel

10. Cholangitis[62] is inflammation of the bile ducts, the vessels that transport bile. The part of cholangitis that means bile is _____. The combining form angi/o means _____. (One *i* in cholangitis is omitted to make pronunciation easier.)

bile

11. Cholangitis is inflammation of the _____ ducts.

12. Cholangiography[63] is x-ray of the bile ducts, usually using a

---

[58] hep″ah ti′tis
[59] hep″ah to meg′ah le
[60] sir ro′sis

[61] hep″ah to tok′sik
[62] ko″lan ji′tis
[63] ko lan″je og′rah fe

cholangiogram[64]	contrast agent. The record of the bile ducts produced in cholangiography is called a _____.
	13. The combining form cyst/o means bladder or sac. Whenever you see *cholecyst* in a word, you will know that it means
gallbladder	_____.
cholecystitis[65]	14. Inflammation of the gallbladder is _____.
gallbladder	15. Cholecystography[66] is examination of the _____ by x-ray study.
gallstones	16. Sometimes gallstones are seen on x-ray. Chole/lith/iasis[67] is the presence of _____ in the gallbladder.
pancreatolith[68]	17. Stones can also form in the pancreas. Write a word that means pancreatic stone: _____
pancreatolithectomy[69]	18. Excision of a pancreatic stone is _____.
salivary glands	19. Saliva is produced by the salivary glands. Sialography[70] is x-ray examination of the _____ _____ and ducts.
stone	20. Sialo/lith/iasis[71] is the presence of a salivary _____.
digestion	21. The suffix -pepsia means _____.
bad	22. If eupepsia[72] is good or normal digestion, dyspepsia[73] is _____ digestion.

---

[64] ko lan′je o gram
[65] ko″le sis ti′tis
[66] ko″le sis tog′rah fe
[67] ko″le lĭ thi′ah sis
[68] pan″kre at′o lith

[69] pan″kre ah to lĭ thek′ to me
[70] si″ah log′rah fe
[71] si″ah lo li thi′ah sis
[72] u pep′se ah
[73] dis pep′se ah

viscera	23. The term *viscera*[74] refers to large internal organs enclosed within a cavity, especially the abdominal organs. Thus, many of the digestive organs are viscera. Write the term that means large internal organs within the abdominal cavity: _____
periton/o	24. Peritoneum is the membrane that surrounds the viscera and lines the abdominal cavity. The peritoneum holds the viscera in position. The combining form for peritoneum is _____.
peritonitis[75]	25. Inflammation of the peritoneum is _____.

TERMS PERTAINING TO SURGICAL PROCEDURES

appendectomy (append/o, appendix, + -ectomy, excision): removal of the vermiform appendix. It is removed when acutely infected to prevent peritonitis, which can occur if the appendix ruptures.

cholecystectomy[76] (cholecyst/o, gallbladder): surgical removal of the gallbladder. Exploration of the common bile duct is often performed during cholecystectomy. In this situation cholangiography (chol/e, bile, + angi/o, vessel, + -graphy, recording) is performed. The biliary vessels are injected with dye and x-rays are taken to determine if stones are present.

colostomy[77] (col/o, colon, + -stomy, artificial opening): creation of a surgical passage through the abdominal wall into the colon. It is performed when the feces cannot pass through the colon and out through the anus.

gastrectomy[78] (gastr/o, stomach): surgical removal of all or part of the stomach

gastrostomy[79]: surgical creation of a new opening into the stomach through the abdominal wall. This allows the insertion of a synthetic feeding tube and is performed when the patient cannot eat normally.

hemorrhoidectomy[80]: removal of hemorrhoids by any of several means, including surgery

ileostomy[81]: creation of a surgical passage through the abdominal wall into the ileum. An ileostomy is necessary when the large intestine has been removed. Fecal material from the ileum drains through an opening called a *stoma* into a bag worn on the abdomen.

liver biopsy: removal of tissue from the liver for pathologic examination. A **percutaneous**[82] liver biopsy is removal of liver tissue by puncturing the skin overlying the liver with a needle. This is considered to be a closed biopsy. (Percutaneous is derived from per-, through, + cutane/o, skin, + -ous, pertaining to.) An open liver biopsy involves

---

[74] vis′er ah
[75] per″ĭ to ni′tis
[76] ko″le sis tek′to me
[77] ko los′to me
[78] gas trek′to me

[79] gas tros′to me
[80] hem″o roid ek′to me
[81] il″e os′to me
[82] per″ku ta′ne us

incision of the abdominal wall to remove liver tissue for pathologic examination.

vagotomy[83] (vag/o, vagus nerve, + -tomy, incision): resection (partial excision) of portions of the vagus nerve near the stomach. This procedure is performed to decrease the amount of gastric juices by severing the nerve (vagus nerve) that controls their release.

EXERCISE III *Write letters in the blanks to correctly complete each word.*

1. Removal of all or part of the stomach is __ __ __ __ __ectomy.
2. Creation of a surgical passage through the abdominal wall into the colon is called a __ __ __ __stomy.
3. Resection of the vagus nerve is __ __ __ __tomy.
4. Removal of the gallbladder is __ __ __ __ __ __ __ __ __ectomy.
5. An __ __ __ __ __ __ __ __ __ is creation of a surgical passage through the abdominal wall into the ileum.
6. Surgical creation of a new opening into the stomach is called __ __ __ __ __ __ __ __ __ __ __.

(Check your answers.)

DISEASES, DISORDERS, AND DIAGNOSTIC TERMS

The Mouth

cheilitis[84] (cheil/o, lip, + -itis, inflammation): inflammation of the lip

gingivitis[85] (gingiv/o, gum): inflammation of the gums

glossitis[86] (gloss/o, tongue): inflammation of the tongue. The tongue is painful, and sometimes covered with ulcers, and swallowing is difficult.

stomatitis[87] (stomat/o, mouth): inflammation of the mouth

The Esophagus

dysphagia[88] (dys-, painful or difficult, + phag/o, eat, + -ia, condition): inability to swallow or difficulty in swallowing. This condition is often associated with such disorders as paralysis, constriction, or spasm of the esophageal muscles.

esophagitis[89] (esophag/o, esophagus): inflammation of the esophagus

The Stomach

gastrocele[90] (gastr/o, stomach, + -cele, hernia): herniation of the stomach. A common type of gastrocele is a **hiatus**[91] (or **hiatal**[92]) **hernia,** protrusion

---

[83] va got′o me
[84] ki li′tis
[85] jin″ji vi′tis
[86] glos si′tis
[87] sto mah ti′tis

[88] dis fa′je ah
[89] ĕ sof″ah ji′tis
[90] gas′tro sēl
[91] hi a′tus
[92] hi a′tal

of a structure through the opening in the diaphragm that allows passage for the esophagus. Often the protruding structure is part of the stomach.

gastroenteritis[93] (enter/o, intestine): inflammation of the stomach and the intestinal tract

gastroscopy[94] (-scopy, visual examination): examination of the interior of the stomach using an endoscope.[95] An endoscope (endo-, inside, + -scope, instrument used for viewing) is a special device consisting of a tube and optical system, and it is used to inspect body organs such as the stomach. Gastroscopy is a type of endoscopy,[96] visual inspection of a body cavity using an endoscope.

ulcer[97]: a lesion of the mucous membrane, accompanied by sloughing (shedding) of dead tissue

The Intestines

appendicitis (append/o, appendix, + -itis, inflammation): inflammation of the vermiform appendix

colitis[98] (col/o, colon): inflammation of the colon

diverticulitis[99] (diverticul/o, diverticulum[100]): inflammation of a diverticulum in the intestinal tract, especially in the colon, causing stagnation or lack of movement of feces and pain. If diverticulitis is severe a **diverticulectomy**[101] is performed. A **diverticulum** (pl., diverticula) is a small sac or pouch in the wall of an organ.

duodenal ulcer: an ulcer of the duodenum. Bleeding is sometimes present with this type of ulcer. Perforation can occur, which can lead to peritonitis (periton/o, peritoneum).

duodenitis[102]: inflammation of the duodenum

enterostasis[103] (enter/o, intestine, + -stasis, stopping): stoppage or delay in the passage of food through the intestine

gastrointestinal (GI) series: the use of contrast agents and x-ray to evaluate the gastrointestinal tract. In an upper GI study the patient drinks barium sulfate, which is radiopaque. X-rays are taken as the barium passes through the esophagus, stomach, and small intestine. The large intestine is evaluated in a lower GI study.

hemorrhoids: masses of veins in the anal canal that are unnaturally distended and lie just inside or outside the rectum. They are often accompanied by pain, itching, and bleeding.

proctoscopy[104] (proct/o, anus or rectum): inspection of the rectum and lower part of the intestine using a proctoscope

sigmoidoscopy: examination of the sigmoid colon using a sigmoidoscope

The Gallbladder

cholecystitis (cholecyst/o, gallbladder): inflammation of the gallbladder

cholecystography (-graphy, recording): x-ray examination of the gallbladder after the bile is rendered opaque

cholelithiasis (chol/e, gall or bile, + lith/o, stone, + -iasis, condition) formation or presence

---

[93] gas"tro en ter i'tis
[94] gas tros'ko pe
[95] en'do skōp
[96] en dos'ko pe
[97] ul'ser
[98] ko li'tis

[99] di"ver tik u li'tis
[100] di"ver tik' u lum
[101] di"ver tik"u lek'to me
[102] du"od ĕ ni'tis
[103] en"ter o sta'sis
[104] prok tos'ko pe

of gallstones in the gallbladder or common bile duct

cholestasis[105] (-stasis, stopping): stoppage of bile excretion

The Liver

cirrhosis: a chronic liver disease characterized by marked degeneration of liver cells

hepatitis (hepat/o, liver): inflammation of the liver

hepatomegaly (-megaly, enlargement): enlargement of the liver

The Pancreas

diabetes: a general term for diseases characterized by excessive urination, but it usually refers to **diabetes mellitus.** Diabetes mellitus is a disorder of carbohydrate metabolism characterized by hyperglycemia resulting from inadequate production or utilization of insulin.

hypoglycemia (hypo-, below normal, + glyc/o, sugar, + -emia, blood): a condition in which the blood glucose level is abnormally low. It can be caused by excessive production of insulin by the pancreas or by excessive injection of insulin.

pancreatitis[106]: inflammation of the pancreas

EXERCISE IV   *Circle the correct answer to complete each sentence.*

1. The presence of gallstones in the gallbladder or common bile duct is (cholecystitis, cholecystography, cholelithiasis, cholestasis).
2. One type of liver disease is (cirrhosis, diverticulitis, dysphagia, splenomegaly).
3. A lesion of a mucous membrane accompanied by sloughing of dead tissue is (dysphagia, diverticulitis, a hemorrhoid, an ulcer).
4. Hiatal hernia is one type of (enterostasis, esophagitis, gastrocele, peptic ulcer).
5. Inflammation of the tongue is (cheilitis, gingivitis, glossitis, stomatitis).
6. A disorder of carbohydrate metabolism that results from inadequate production or utilization of insulin is commonly called (celiac disease, diabetes, dyspepsia, hypoglycemia).
7. Varicose veins of the anal canal are called (diverticula, hemorrhoids, hepatitis, hepatomegaly).
8. Sigmoidoscopy is examination of part of the (esophagus, large intestine, liver, small intestine).

Be sure that you recognize the meaning of the following word parts that have been introduced in this chapter.

---

[105] ko"le sta'sis   [106] pan"kre ah ti'tis

ADDITIONAL WORD PARTS

Word Part	Meaning
de-	down, from, reversing or removing
-eal	pertaining to
-emia	blood
ur/o	urine or urinary tract
vag/o	vagus nerve

EXERCISE V

Write a letter in each of the blank spaces to complete the following sentences.

1. Inflammation of the esophagus is __ __ __ __ __ __ __itis.
2. Inflammation of the stomach and intestinal tract is gastro__ __ __ __ __itis.
3. Stoppage or delay in the passage of food through the intestine is entero__ __ __ __ __ __.
4. Inspection of the stomach using an endoscope is called __ __ __ __ __ __scopy.
5. Inflammation of the vermiform appendix is called __ __ __ __ __ __ __ __itis.
6. Removal of the gallbladder is __ __ __ __ __ __ __ __ __ec-tomy.
7. Inflammation of the liver is __ __ __ __ __itis.
8. Abnormally low blood sugar is hypo__ __ __ __ __ __ __ __.

(Check your answers.)

Comprehensive Review Exercises

WORK THE FOLLOWING EXERCISES TO TEST YOUR UNDERSTANDING OF THE MATERIAL IN CHAPTER 8. IT IS BEST TO DO ALL THE REVIEW EXERCISES BEFORE CHECKING YOUR ANSWERS.

A. Match the underlined word parts in the left column with their meanings in the right column.

_____ 1. <u>stoma</u>titis   A. bile
_____ 2. ped<u>od</u>ontics   B. digestion
_____ 3. hep<u>a</u>titis   C. intestines

(This exercise continues on the next page.)

____	4. sialography	D. lip
____	5. dyspepsia	E. liver
____	6. gastrectomy	F. mouth
____	7. cheilitis	G. salivary glands
____	8. glossitis	H. stomach
____	9. enterostasis	I. teeth
____	10. cholelithiasis	J. tongue

B. Using word parts you have learned, write letters in the blanks to correctly complete each sentence.

1. A term that means under the tongue is hypo__ __ __ __ __al.

2. The branch of dentistry that specializes in the tissue that invests and supports the teeth is peri__ __ __ __ __ics.

3. The branch of medicine that specializes in the stomach, intestines, and associated structures is gastro__ __ __ __ __ __-logy.

4. A physician who specializes in diseases of the anus, rectum, and colon is a __ __ __ __ __ __logist.

5. A chronic liver disease characterized by marked degeneration of the liver is __ __ __ __ __osis.

6. Inflammation of the bile ducts is __ __ __ __angitis.

7. A disorder of carbohydrate metabolism that results from inadequate production or utilization of insulin is __ __ __ __ __ __ __ __ mellitus.

8. Excision of a pancreatic stone is pancreato__ __ __ __ectomy.

9. Creation of an opening onto the abdominal surface from the colon is a colo__ __ __ __ __.

10. Inflammation of the lip is __ __ __ __ __ __ __ __ __ __.

C. Circle the correct answer for each of the following.

1. A condition that results when the output of body fluid exceeds fluid intake is (achlorhydria, dehydration, enterostasis, peristalsis).

2. Which of the following is *not* part of the small intestine? (cecum, duodenum, jejunum, ileum)

3. Which of the following is *not* considered an accessory organ of the digestive system? (gallbladder, liver, salivary gland, spleen)

4. Another name for the gum is (gingiva, peristalsis, pylorus, stoma).

5. Washing out of the stomach is called (gastralgia, gastric lavage, gastrodynia, stomal irrigation).

6. The presence of stones in the gallbladder or common duct is (cholangiography, cholecystitis, cholecystography, cholelithiasis).

7. Which of the following is *not* generally characteristic of untreated diabetes mellitus? (glycosuria, hyperglycemia, jaundice, polyuria)

8. Large internal organs of the body are called (anastoma, melena, peritoneum, viscera).

9. Removal of liver tissue by puncturing the skin overlying the liver with a needle is called (open, resection, percutaneous, wedge) liver biopsy.

10. A procedure performed to decrease the amount of gastric juices by severing the nerves that control their release is a (cholecystectomy, colon resection, gastrectomy, vagotomy).

11. Inablity to swallow or difficulty in swallowing is (diverticulitis, dyspepsia, dysphagia, lithiasis).

12. Inflammation of a small sac or pouch in the intestinal tract that causes stagnation of feces and pain is (colitis, diverticulitis, duodenitis, hemorrhoids).

13. A GI series refers to the use of contrast agents to evaluate the (gallbladder, gastrointestinal tract, pancreas, salivary glands).

14. Cirrhosis is a chronic disease of the (gallbladder, liver, pancreas, stomach).

15. Gastrocele means herniation of the (gallbladder, large intestine, liver, stomach).

D. Write the medical term for which each meaning is given:

1. loss of appetite for food _____

2. excessive vomiting _____

3. pertaining to the esophagus _____

4. pertaining to the stomach _____

5. stoppage of bile excretion _____

6. enlargement of the liver _____

7. inflammation of the gallbladder _____

8. removal of the vermiform appendix _____

9. inflammation of the gums _____

10. x-ray examination of the gallbladder _____

11. inflammation of the liver _____

12. abnormally low blood sugar level _____

9

The Urinary System

OBJECTIVES

After completing Chapter 9, you will be able to

1. Write the meaning of the word parts pertaining to the urinary system that are presented in this chapter and choose their correct meanings when presented with several answers.
2. Analyze terms related to the urinary system, select the appropriate response when presented with several answers, and write the term when presented with its definition.

OUTLINE

EXCRETION OF BODY WASTES
ELIMINATION OF WASTES BY THE KIDNEYS
STRUCTURE OF THE URINARY TRACT
TERMS PERTAINING TO SURGICAL PROCEDURES
DISEASES, DISORDERS, AND DIAGNOSTIC TERMS
THE URINE
COMPREHENSIVE REVIEW EXERCISES

EXCRETION OF BODY WASTES

The body produces wastes that are eliminated by the process of **excretion.**[1] There are several ways in which the body eliminates waste. The lungs and other parts of the respiratory system eliminate carbon dioxide, the digestive system rids the body of solid waste, and the skin eliminates wastes through perspiration. Many waste products resulting from the metabolism of food are eliminated through **urination,**[2] the act of voiding urine. The kidneys, ureters,[3] bladder, and urethra[4] comprise the **urinary**[5] **system.** The organs and ducts participating in the secretion and elimination of urine are called the **urinary tract.**

ELIMINATION OF WASTES BY THE KIDNEYS

Excretion of waste products by the kidneys is vital for good health. **Urea**[6] (ur/o, urine) is the final product of protein metabolism and is the chief nitrogenous waste present in urine. **Uremia**[7] (ur/o + -emia, blood) is a toxic condition associated with renal insufficiency or renal failure. The term **renal**[8] (ren/o, kidney) is a commonly used adjective that means pertaining to the kidney. **Renal insufficiency** (in-, not) is the reduced ability of the kidney to perform its functions. Acute renal failure is failure of the kidney to perform its essential functions, and is a critical situation. Kidney dialysis or **hemodialysis**[9] (hem/o, blood) is required if the kidneys fail to remove waste products from the blood. Kidney dialysis is the process of diffusing blood through a membrane to remove toxic materials and maintain proper chemical balance. **Peritoneal dialysis**[10] is an alternative to hemodialysis (peritoneal is derived from periton/o, peritoneum, + -eal, pertaining to). The peritoneum is the membrane that covers the large internal organs of the abdominal cavity and lines that cavity. In peritoneal dialysis the dialyzing solution is introduced into and removed from the peritoneal cavity.

Diuretic[11] means increasing urination or an agent that causes increased urination. Some common substances such as tea, coffee, and water act as diuretics. Increased or excessive urination is called either **diuresis**[12] or **polyuria**[13] (poly-, many, + ur/o, urine, + -ia, condition).

---

[1] eks kre'shun
[2] u"rĭ na'shun
[3] u re'terz
[4] u re'thrah
[5] u'rĭ ner"e
[6] u re'ah
[7] u re'me ah

[8] re'nal
[9] he"mo di al'ĭ sis
[10] per"ĭ to ne'al di al'ĭ sis
[11] di"u ret'ik
[12] di"u re'sis
[13] pol"e u're ah

Urology[14] (ur/o, urine or urinary tract, + -logy, science of) is the branch of medicine concerned with the male genital tract and the urinary tracts of both sexes. A **urologist**[15] is a physician who specializes in the practice of urology.

STRUCTURE OF THE URINARY TRACT

The urinary system is composed of two kidneys, a ureter for each kidney, a bladder, and a urethra (Fig. 9–1).

The **kidneys** have the shape of kidney beans (hence, the name of the bean). They are situated at the back of the abdominal cavity, one on each side of the spinal column. A kidney contains approximately

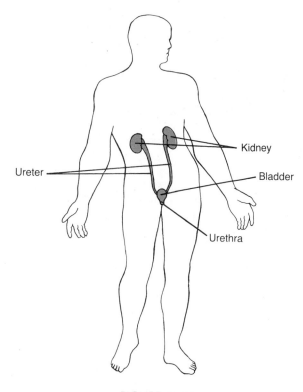

FIGURE 9–1

The urinary system in relation to the body outline. (From Leonard, P.C.: *Building a Medical Vocabulary*. 2nd ed. Philadelphia, W.B. Saunders, 1988.)

---

[14] u rol'o je   [15] u rol'o jist

1,000,000 microscopic nephrons,[16] its functional units. Each kidney functions independently of the other one.

Urine leaves the kidney by way of the **ureter.** Both ureters lead to the **urinary bladder,** where urine is stored. Filling of the bladder with urine produces the desire to urinate. Voluntary control prevents urine from being released. When this control is removed, urine is expelled through a canal called the urethra.

EXERCISE I

Use one of the following words to correctly complete each sentence.

diuresis   hemodialysis   urea
diuretic   nephron   uremia

1. Diffusing blood through a membrane to remove wastes and maintain proper chemical balance is called _____.
2. An agent that causes increased urination is a _____.
3. Excessive or increased urination is _____.
4. _____ is a toxic condition of the body that is associated with renal failure.
5. The functional unit of the kidney is the _____.
6. A major waste product found in urine is _____.

EXERCISE II

Match the terms in the left column with their meanings in the right column.

_____ 1. urinary bladder
_____ 2. nephron
_____ 3. peritoneum
_____ 4. ureter
_____ 5. urethra

A. the complete functional unit of the kidney
B. where urine is stored until urination
C. membrane that lines the abdominal cavity
D. tube through which urine passes from the kidney
E. tubular passage by which urine is discharged from the bladder

(Check your answers with the solutions in the back of the book.)

Combining forms for major structures of the urinary system are presented in the following list. Commit these to **memory.**

---

[16] nef'ronz

WORD PARTS PERTAINING TO STRUCTURES OF THE URINARY SYSTEM

Combining Form	Name of Structure
cyst/o	bladder (sometimes, cyst or sac)
glomerul/o	glomerulus[17] (filtering structure of the kidney)
nephr/o, ren/o	kidney
pyel/o	renal pelvis (reservoir in the kidney that collects the urine)
ureter/o	ureter
urethr/o	urethra

PROGRAMMED LEARNING

Remember to cover the answers in the left column and then slide the card down to check each answer after you have written it in the blank.

nephr/o, ren/o	1. The two combining forms that mean the kidney are _____ and _____.
kidney	2. Nephro/malacia[18] is softening of the _____.
enlargement	3. Nephro/megaly[19] is _____ of one or both kidneys.
unilateral[21]	4. Bilateral[20] nephromegaly is enlargement of both kidneys. Lateral pertains to a side. Bi/lateral (bi-, two) means pertaining to two sides—in other words, both sides. You previously learned two prefixes (mono- and uni-) that mean *one*. Monolateral is *not* commonly used. Use the other prefix for *one* to write a term that means pertaining to one side: _____
	5. Nephromegaly and many other structural abnormalities of the kidneys can be observed by nephro/sonography,[22] which is the

---

[17] glo mer′u lus
[18] nef″ro mah la′she ah
[19] nef″ro meg′ah le

[20] bi lat′er al
[21] u″nĭ lat′er al
[22] nef″ro so nog′rah fe

kidneys

use of ultrasound to make a record of the kidneys. (Remember that -graphy means the process of recording. A new word part, *son/o*, means sound.) Nephrosonography is the use of ultrasound to make a record of the _____.

---

nephrotomog-raphy[24]

6. Computed tomography[23] is also helpful for visualizing the kidney without surgical invasion. Through a special technique, computed tomography produces a picture of an internal structure as though one were viewing a cross section of the organ. Combine nephr/o and tomography to form a word that means computed tomography of the kidney: _____

---

nephroptosis[25]

7. Remembering that -ptosis means sagging or prolapse, use nephr/o to write a word that means prolapse of a kidney: _____ This is also called a hypermobile (hyper-, excessive) or floating kidney.

---

surgical fixation

8. Nephroptosis can occur when the kidney supports are weakened by a sudden strain or blow, or the defect can be present at birth. Nephroptosis is usually corrected by nephro/pexy,[26] which is _____ _____ of the kidney.

---

stones

9. Nephro/lith/iasis[27] is a condition marked by the presence of kidney _____.

---

renal

10. Nephro/lith[28] is a word, but kidney stones are usually called renal calculi. Notice that *nephr/o* is used more often in building medical terms, but *ren/o* is used to write an adjective that means pertaining to the kidney. Write that adjective: _____

---

kidney

11. Renal is often used as an adjective to identify a particular procedure or part of the kidney. In a renal transplant, the recipient receives a _____ from a donor.

---

[23] to mog′rah fe
[24] nef″ro to mog′rah fe
[25] nef″rop to′sis
[26] nef′ro pek″se
[27] nef″ro li thi′ah sis
[28] nef′ro lith

pelvis

12. The funnel-shaped cavity in the kidney that collects urine is called the renal _____.

renal

13. *Pelvis* means any basin-shaped structure or cavity. Standing alone, pelvis usually refers to the bony structure that serves as a support for the spinal column. When referring to the funnel-shaped cavity of the kidney, however, it is called the _____ pelvis.

pyel/o

14. The combining form for renal pelvis is _____.

15. Use the combining form from the preceding frame to write a word that means inflammation of the renal pelvis:

pyelitis[29]

_____

16. Nephr/itis,[30] also called Bright's disease, is inflammation of the kidney. The most common form of acute nephritis is glomerulo/nephritis,[31] in which glomeruli (plural of glomerulus) of the

kidney

_____ are inflamed.

17. A pyelo/gram[32] is a film produced by x-ray of the

renal pelvis

_____ _____ after injection of a contrast medium. Other parts of the kidney and ureter are also visible. In an intravenous[33] (intra-, within, + ven/o, vein, + -ous, pertaining to) pyelogram, radiopaque material is injected into a vein. X-rays taken while the material passes through the urinary tract provide information about the structure and function of the kidney, ureter, and bladder.

18. The combining form cyst/o is used to form words pertaining to the urinary bladder, or to a cyst or sac. Cyst/ic[34] has several meanings, including pertaining to a cyst, pertaining to the gall-bladder, and pertaining to the urinary _____. The

bladder

rest of the sentence must usually be read to determine the intended meaning of the word *cystic*.

---

[29] pi″ĕ li′tis
[30] nĕ fri′tis
[31] glo mer″u lo nĕ fri′tis

[32] pi′ĕ lo gram
[33] in″trah ve′nus
[34] sis′tik

bladder

19. Used alone, *bladder* usually refers to the urinary bladder. Cysto/scopy[35] is examination of the urinary bladder. In this procedure, an instrument is passed through the urethra and into the _____.

cystoscope[36]

20. The lining of the bladder is examined by special lenses, mirrors, and a light. The instrument used in cystoscopy is a _____.

cystitis[37]

21. Inflammation of the bladder is _____.

nephritis

22. Sometimes people say they have a kidney infection when they actually have cystitis, a more common type of urinary tract infection. Inflammation of the kidney is _____.

ureter

23. Two tubular passageways that convey urine to and from the bladder are the ureters and the urethra, respectively. Uretero/plasty[38] is surgical repair of a _____.

urethral[40]

24. Ureteral[39] pertains to a ureter. Use ureteral as a model to write a word that means pertaining to the urethra: _____.

uremia

25. Uremia is a toxic condition associated with renal insufficiency or renal failure. Urea, the chief nitrogen-containing waste product of protein metabolism, is not properly removed from the blood by the kidneys in uremia. Write the term that refers to the presence of nitrogen-containing waste in the blood: _____.

urine
blood

26. In analyzing the parts of ur/emia, ur/o means _____ and -emia means _____. The meaning of uremia cannot be interpreted literally from its word parts, so pay particular attention to its meaning! (It might help to think of *urea in the blood,* but you also need to remember that uremia is a toxic condition associated with renal insufficiency or failure.)

27. Another medical term that uses word parts for *urine* and *blood* is

---

[35] sis tos′ko pe
[36] sis′to skōp
[37] sis ti′tis

[38] u re′ter o plas″te
[39] u re′ter al
[40] u re′thral

hematuria

hemat/uria.[41] In this term, one must again decide on the correct meaning. Hematuria means blood in the urine. Write the medical term that means blood in the urine: _____

28. It is easy to confuse the two medical terms you just learned in the last three frames. For practice, write the terms for the following: a toxic condition associated with renal failure: _____
blood in the urine: _____

uremia
hematuria

EXERCISE III

Match the combining forms in the left column with their meanings in the right column (the choices on the right may be used more than once).

_____ 1. cyst/o   A. bladder
_____ 2. nephr/o   B. kidney
_____ 3. pyel/o   C. renal pelvis
_____ 4. ren/o   D. ureter
_____ 5. ureter/o   E. urethra
_____ 6. urethr/o

EXERCISE IV

Using word parts you have learned, write letters in the blanks to correctly complete each sentence.

1. Softening of the kidney is __ __ __ __ __ __malacia.
2. Pertaining to the urethra is __ __ __ __ __ __al.
3. The term for enlargement of one or both kidneys is nephro- __ __ __ __ __ __.
4. Pertaining to a ureter is __ __ __ __ __ __ __ __.
5. Surgical fixation of a prolapsed kidney is nephro __ __ __ __.
6. An acute nephritis in which the glomeruli of the kidney are inflamed is __ __ __ __ __ __ __ __ __nephritis.
7. Inflammation of the renal pelvis is __ __ __ __ __ __ __ __.
8. The presence of kidney stones is nephro __ __ __ __iasis.
9. Inflammation of the bladder is __ __ __ __ __ __ __ __.
10. The term for examination of the bladder is __ __ __ __ __ __ __ __ __.

(Check your answers.)

_____

[41] hem"ah tu're ah

TERMS PERTAINING TO SURGICAL PROCEDURES

cystostomy[42] (cyst/o, bladder, + -stomy, new opening): surgical creation of a temporary opening into the bladder

lithotripsy[43] (lith/o, stone, + -tripsy, surgical crushing): surgical crushing of a stone. A **lithotrite**[44] is an instrument for crushing bladder stones.

nephrolithotomy[45] (nephr/o, kidney, + -tomy, incision): incision of the kidney for removal of a kidney stone (removal of the stone is implied in this term)

nephropexy (-pexy, surgical fixation): surgical attachment of a prolapsed kidney

nephrostomy[46] (-stomy, artificial opening): creation of a new opening into the renal pelvis of the kidney (the opening into the renal pelvis is implied). This procedure is usually done to drain urine from the kidney.

percutaneous bladder biopsy: removal of tissue from the bladder using a needle inserted through the skin overlying the bladder; done for diagnostic purposes (percutaneous[47] is derived from per-, through, + cutane/o, skin, + -ous, pertaining to)

percutaneous renal biopsy: removal of tissue from the kidney using needle puncture of the skin and tissue overlying the kidney; done for diagnostic purposes

pyelolithotomy[48] (pyel/o, renal pelvis, +lith/o, stone, + -tomy, incision): surgical incision of the kidney to remove a stone from the renal pelvis (removal of the stone is implied)

pyelostomy[49] (-stomy, new opening): surgical formation of a new opening into the renal pelvis

DISEASES, DISORDERS, AND DIAGNOSTIC TERMS

anuria (an-, without, + -uria, urine or urination): absence of urination or production of less than 100 ml of urine/day

blood urea nitrogen (BUN): a substance in the blood, the level of which provides a rough estimate of kidney function. An increase in the BUN concentration usually indicates that the kidneys are not removing enough waste urea from the blood.

catheterization[50]: passage of a tubular, flexible instrument (catheter[51]) into a body channel or cavity, usually done for withdrawal or introduction of fluid

cystitis (cyst/o, bladder, + -itis, inflammation): inflammation of the urinary bladder

cystocele[52] (-cele, hernia): a bladder hernia that protrudes into the vagina

cystoscopy (-scopy, visual examination): examination inside the bladder with an instrument (**cystoscope**) introduced through the urethra

glomerulonephritis (glomerul/o, glomerulus, + nephr/o, kidney): a type of nephritis in which the glomeruli of the kidney are inflamed. It can be acute or chronic, and frequently occurs after infection elsewhere in the body, especially in the upper respiratory tract.

intravenous pyelogram: x-ray of the urinary tract after injection of a radiopaque material into a vein

nephrolithiasis (lith/o, stone, + -iasis, condition): the presence of stones in the kidney

nephromalacia (-malacia, softening): abnormal renal softening

nephromegaly (-megaly, enlarged): enlargement of one or both kidneys

---

[42] sis tos'to me
[43] lith'o trip"se
[44] lith'o trīt
[45] nef"ro lǐ thot'o me
[46] ně fros'to me
[47] per"ku ta'ne us

[48] pi"ě lo lǐ thot'o me
[49] pi"ě los'to me
[50] kath"ě ter i za'shun
[51] kath'ě ter
[52] sis'to sēl

nephroptosis (-ptosis, prolapse): prolapse or downward displacement of the kidney

nephrosis[53] (-osis, condition): a condition in which there are degenerative changes in the kidneys but no inflammation

nephrosonography (son/o, sound, + -graphy, recording): ultrasonic scanning of the kidney

nephrotomography (tom/o, cut): computed tomography of the kidney

nephrotoxic[54]: destructive to kidney tissue

polycystic[55] **kidney disease** (poly-, many, + cyst/o, cyst, + -ic, pertaining to): a hereditary disorder characterized by hundreds of fluid-filled cysts throughout both kidneys

polyp[56]: a tumor found on a mucosal surface, such as the inner lining of the bladder

polyuria: excessive secretion and discharge of urine; also called diuresis

pyelitis (pyel/o, renal pelvis): inflammation of the renal pelvis

pyelogram (-gram, record): a record produced by x-ray of the urinary tract after intravenous injection of radiopaque material

pyuria[57] (py/o, pus, + -uria, urine): pus in the urine

renal failure: failure of the kidney to perform its essential functions

retrograde pyelography: x-ray of the renal pelvis and ureter after injection of a contrast medium into the renal pelvis. In this procedure the contrast material is injected through catheters that are introduced into the ureters. (The prefix retro- means behind or backward. The use of retrograde pyelography provides an alternative to intravenous pyelography [IVP] for viewing the renal pelvis and ureters. In IVP, the contrast medium flows through the renal pelvis and ureters after reaching the kidney by way of the bloodstream. In retrograde pyelography, contrast medium is introduced through the ureter, and could be considered backward or in the opposite manner of IVP.)

urinary incontinence[58] (in-, not): inability to hold urine in the bladder

urinary retention: inability to empty the bladder

urinary tract infection (UTI): an infection of the urinary tract

voiding cystourethrogram[59] (cyst/o, bladder, + urethr/o, urethra): an x-ray record of the bladder and urethra. After the bladder has been filled with a contrast medium, x-rays are taken while the patient is expelling urine.

EXERCISE V

Write the meaning of each underlined word part in the blank spaces.

1. <u>cyst</u>itis _____
2. <u>glomerulonephr</u>itis _____
3. <u>nephr</u>omalacia _____
4. poly<u>cyst</u>ic kidney _____
5. <u>pyel</u>itis _____
6. py<u>uria</u> _____
7. <u>litho</u>trite _____
8. nephro<u>son</u>ography _____
9. <u>renal</u> _____
10. cysto<u>urethro</u>gram _____

---

[53] ně fro'sis
[54] nef″ro tox'sik
[55] pol″e sis'tik
[56] pol'ip

[57] pi u're ah
[58] in kon'tĭ nens
[59] sis″to u re'thro gram

EXERCISE VI   *Circle the correct answer to complete each sentence.*

1. An inability to empty the bladder is called (cystitis, urinary incontinence, urinary retention, urinary tract infection).
2. The absence of urination is (anuria, diuresis, pyuria, polyuria).
3. Examination inside the bladder using a special instrument passed through the urethra is (catheterization, cystoscopy, cystostomy, urethrogram).
4. A condition of degenerative changes in the kidneys that does not involve inflammation is called (nephritis, nephromegaly, nephrosis, nephrostomy).
5. A record produced by x-ray of the urinary tract after injection of a radiopaque material is called an intravenous (nephroptosis, nephrosonogram, nephrotomogram, pyelogram).
6. Surgical crushing of a stone is (lithotriptor, lithotomy, lithotripsy, nephrolithotomy).
7. Creation of a new opening into the renal pelvis is (nephropexy, nephroptosis, nephrostomy, percutaneous renal biopsy).
8. In pyelolithotomy, a stone is removed from the (bladder, renal pelvis, ureter, urethra).

(Check your answers.)

THE URINE   **Urinalysis**[60] is the examination of urine specimens by laboratory tests. Many substances for which urine is tested are not found in a normal urine specimen — for example, sugar, protein, and blood. The presence of one of these substances in urine is called **glycosuria**[61] (glycos/o, sugar, + -uria, urine), **proteinuria**,[62] and **hematuria** (hemat/o, blood), respectively. The term **albuminuria**[63] is sometimes used instead of proteinuria when there is a very high concentration of albumin, one type of protein, in the urine. **Pyuria** (py/o, pus) is the presence of pus in the urine.

In addition to combining forms that pertain to the urinary system, a few other word parts have been used that might be new to you. They are presented in the list that follows. Be sure that you **recognize their meanings**.

---

[60] u″rĭ nal′ĭ sis   [62] pro″te in u′re ah
[61] gli″ko su′re ah   [63] al″bu mĭ nu′re ah

**ADDITIONAL
COMBINING FORMS**

Combining Form	Meaning
albumin/o	albumin
-eal	pertaining to
hemat/o, hem/o, -emia	blood
periton/o	peritoneum
son/o	sound
ur/o	urine or urinary tract
-uria	urine or urination

EXERCISE VII

Match the terms in the left column, which indicate the abnormal presence of various substances in the urine, with the substance in the right column.

_____ 1. albuminuria   A. blood
_____ 2. glycosuria   B. protein
_____ 3. hematuria   C. pus
_____ 4. pyuria   D. sugar

Comprehensive Review Exercises

WORK THE FOLLOWING EXERCISES TO TEST YOUR UNDERSTANDING OF
THE MATERIAL IN CHAPTER 9. IT IS BEST TO DO ALL THE REVIEW EXERCISES
BEFORE CHECKING YOUR ANSWERS.

A. Complete the following by writing terms pertaining to the urinary system in the blank spaces.

The organs and ducts participating in the secretion and elimination of urine are called the (1) _____ tract. Urine leaves the kidney by way of the (2) _____. Urine is stored in the (3) _____ until it is excreted. The canal by which urine leaves the bladder is the (4) _____.

The chief nitrogenous waste product found in the urine is
(5) _____. Acute renal failure can lead to a toxic
condition in which these nitrogenous substances are not excreted
and therefore remain in the blood. This toxic condition is called
(6) _____.

B. Match the terms in the left column with their meanings in the right column (not all selections will be used).

_____ 1. diuretic
_____ 2. polyuria
_____ 3. polyp
_____ 4. pyuria
_____ 5. urinalysis
_____ 6. urinary inconti-
nence
_____ 7. urinary reten-
tion

A. common laboratory examination to determine substances in urine
B. growth found on mucosal surfaces
C. infection of the urinary tract
D. inability to empty the bladder
E. excessive urination
F. agent that causes increased urination
G. pus in the urine
H. sugar in the urine
I. inability to hold urine in the bladder

C. Write letters in the blanks to correctly complete each word.

1. Softening of the kidney is __ __ __ __ __ __ malacia.
2. Visualization of the kidney using ultrasound is nephro-
__ __ __ __ __ __ __ __ __ __.
3. Passage of a tubular, flexible instrument into a body channel or cavity for withdrawal or introduction of fluid is called __ __ __ __ __ __ __ __ ization.
4. A type of nephritis in which the glomeruli of the kidney are inflamed is __ __ __ __ __ __ __ __ __ nephritis.
5. A hereditary disorder characterized by the presence of hundreds of fluid-filled cysts throughout both kidneys is called __ __ __ __ __ __ __ __ __ __ kidney disease.
6. The instrument used in cystoscopy is a cysto __ __ __ __ __.
7. Incision of the kidney to remove a calculus is nephro- __ __ __ __ __ tomy.

8. A film of the kidneys and ureters produced after injection of a radiopaque material into a vein is called an intravenous __ __ __ __ __gram.

9. A bladder hernia that protrudes into the vagina is a __ __ __ __ __cele.

10. The presence of protein in the urine is protein __ __ __ __.

D. Write the meaning of each underlined word part in the blank spaces.

1. <u>pyelo</u>stomy _____

2. py<u>uria</u> _____

3. <u>hemo</u>dialysis _____

4. <u>litho</u>trite _____

5. <u>cysto</u>urethrogram _____

E. Circle the correct answer to complete each sentence.

1. Enlargement of one or both kidneys is (diuresis, nephromegaly, nephropexy, nephroptosis).
2. Renal pertains to (the bladder, the kidney, urine, urination).
3. A condition in which there are degenerative, but not inflammatory, changes in the kidneys is (catheterization, nephritis, nephrosis, percutaneous nephrostomy).
4. Surgical incision of the kidney to remove a stone from the renal pelvis is (lithotripsy, lithotrite, pyelolithotomy, ureterolithotomy).
5. Blood in the urine is (albuminuria, hematuria, ketonuria, proteinuria).

F. Write the correct answer in each blank space. The first letter of each word is given as a clue.

1. The branch of medicine concerned with the urinary tract in both sexes and the male genital tract is u_____.

2. Examination of the urinary bladder is c_____.

3. Pertaining to a ureter is u_____.

4. Sugar in the urine is g_____.

5. Destructive to kidney tissue is n_____.

G. Write the medical term for which each meaning is given:

1. pertaining to the kidney _____

2. inflammation of the renal pelvis _____

3. surgical repair of a ureter _____

4. pertaining to the urethra _____

5. absence of urination _____

6. formation of a new opening into the bladder _____

10 The Reproductive System

OBJECTIVES

After completing Chapter 10, you will be able to

1. Write the meaning of the word parts pertaining to the reproductive system and choose their correct meanings when presented with several answers.
2. Analyze terms related to the reproductive system and obstetrics, select the appropriate response when presented with several answers, and write the terms when presented with their definition.
3. Recognize terms related to the sexually transmitted diseases discussed in this chapter and select the correct response when presented with several answers.

OUTLINE

REPRODUCTION
FEMALE GENITALIA
    Terms pertaining to surgical procedures of the female genitalia
    Diseases, disorders, and diagnostic terms pertaining to the
       female genitalia
OBSTETRICS
    Additional terms related to obstetrics
MALE GENITALIA
    Terms pertaining to surgical procedures of the male genitalia
    Diseases, disorders, and diagnostic terms pertaining to the male
      genitalia
SEXUALLY TRANSMITTED DISEASES
COMPREHENSIVE REVIEW EXERCISES

REPRODUCTION

Reproduction is the process by which genetic material is passed from one generation to the next. The male and female reproductive systems can be broadly organized by organs with different functions. For example, the testes[1] and ovaries[2] are called the **gonads**[3] (gon/o means genitals or reproduction), and they function in the production of sperm or ova (eggs). The gonads also secrete important hormones. Ducts transport and receive eggs or sperm and important fluids. Still other reproductive organs produce materials that support the sperm and ova. Reproductive organs, whether male or female, or internal or external, are called the genitals or **genitalia**.[4]

FEMALE GENITALIA

Gynecology[5] is the study of diseases of the female reproductive organs. These include the **ovaries,** which produce ova, the **uterine**[6] or **fallopian**[7] **tubes,** which transport the ova to the **uterus**[8] (womb), the **vagina**[9] (birth canal), and the external organs that constitute the **vulva**[10] (Fig. 10–1).

Two pairs of skin folds, the labia majora[11] and the labia minora,[12] protect the vaginal opening. (Labia is a term that means lips, or structures that resemble lips. Majora and minora refer to major, or larger, and minor, or smaller.) The labia majora and labia minora are part of the vulva, the female external genitalia. **Vulval**[13] and **Vulvar**[14] (vulv/o, vulva, + -al or -ar, pertaining to) are adjectives that mean pertaining to the vulva.

Words that pertain to the vagina often use the adjective **vaginal**[15] (vagin/o, vagina). The uterus provides nourishment from the time the fertilized egg is implanted to the time of birth of the fetus. A **fetus**[16] is the latter stages of the developing young and, in humans, is that time **in utero** after the first 8 weeks. *In utero* means within the uterus (the combining form uter/o means uterus). **Intrauterine**[17] also means within the uterus, and **extrauterine**[18] means outside the uterus (intra- and -extra mean within and outside, respectively). Uterine is a frequently used adjective that pertains to the uterus.

---

[1] tes′tēz

[2] o′vah rēz

[3] go′nadz, gon′adz

[4] jen″ĭ ta′le ah

[5] gi″nĕ kol′o je, jin″ĕ kol′o je

[6] u′ter īn, u′ter in

[7] fal lo′pe an

[8] u′ter us

[9] vah ji′nah

[10] vul′vah

[11] la′be ah ma jor′ah

[12] la′be ah mi nor′ah

[13] vul′val

[14] vul′var

[15] vaj′ĭ nal

[16] fe′tus

[17] in″trah u′ter in

[18] eks″trah u′ter in

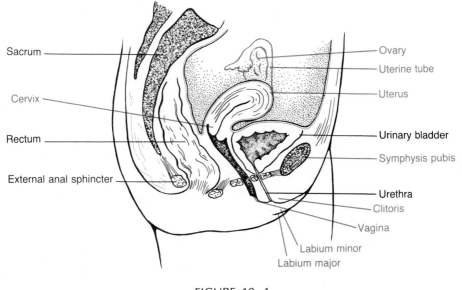

Sacrum · Ovary · Uterine tube · Cervix · Uterus · Rectum · Urinary bladder · Symphysis pubis · External anal sphincter · Urethra · Clitoris · Vagina · Labium minor · Labium major

FIGURE 10–1

Female genitalia *(cross section)*. The sacrum, a triangular bone, forms the base of the vertebral column. The sacrum and anal sphincter (muscle) are labeled to show their positions relative to genital structures, as are the urinary bladder and urethra, structures of the urinary system. (From Leonard, P.C.: *Building a Medical Vocabulary*. 2nd ed. Philadelphia, W.B. Saunders, 1988.)

The **cervix uteri,**[19] commonly called the cervix, is the lowermost cylindric part of the uterus (the combining form cervic/o means the neck or the cervix uteri). The adjective **cervical**[20] pertains either to the neck itself or to the cervix, which is the neck of the uterus. By examining other parts of the word or the way in which it is used, it can usually be decided whether it refers to the neck itself or the cervix. Another combining form that has two meanings is metr/o, which means either measurement or uterine tissue. The tissue that forms the lining of the uterus is called the **endometrium**[21] (endo-, inside, + metr/o, uterine tissue, + -ium, membrane).

A vaginal speculum[22] is used to examine the vagina and the cervix. This instrument can be pushed apart after it is inserted into the vagina to allow visual examination and to collect material for a **Pap smear** (Papanicolaou[23] smear). Early diagnosis of cancer of

[19] ser'viks u'ter i
[20] ser'vĭ kal
[21] en do me'tre um
[22] spek'u lum
[23] pap"ah nik"o la'ooz

the uterus is possible with a Pap smear or Pap test. **Colpocervical**[24] (colp/o, vagina, + cervic/o, cervix) pertains to the vagina and cervix.

The ovaries are located on each side of the uterus. **Ovarian**[25] (ovar/o, ovary) means pertaining to one or both ovaries. Ovaries function in ovulation[26] (the production of ova) and in the production of two important hormones, **estrogen**[27] and **progesterone.**[28] These hormones are responsible for the development and maintenance of secondary sexual characteristics, preparation of the uterus for pregnancy, and development of the mammary (mamm/o, breast) gland.

Menstruation[29] (men/o, month) is the periodic discharge of a bloody fluid from the uterus that occurs at fairly regular intervals from the age of puberty to menopause. The **climacteric,**[30] or **menopause,**[31] marks the end of a woman's reproductive period. Menstruation, also called **menses,**[32] is the sloughing off of the endometrium, which has been prepared to receive a fertilized ovum but is not needed. Menstruation ceases temporarily during pregnancy and breast feeding, and ceases permanently with the onset of menopause (unless hormones are administered). Several menstrual irregularities can occur:

amenorrhea[33] (a-, without, + men/o, month, + -rrhea, discharge): absence of menstrual flow when it is normally expected

dysmenorrhea[34] (dys-, difficult): painful menstruation

menorrhagia[35] (-rrhagia, hemorrhage): excessive flow during menstruation

metrorrhagia[36] (metr/o, uterine tissue): bleeding from the uterus at any time other than during the menstrual period. Translated literally, metrorrhagia means hemorrhage from the uterus. Menstruation, normal menstrual flow, contains the word part men/o, which means month (men/o is used in the words menses and menstruation). You will need to remember that metrorrhagia is abnormal bleeding that is *not* associated with menstruation.

Several combining forms have been introduced. These are presented in the following list, along with a few additional word parts related to the female genitalia. Be sure that you **memorize** the following word parts and their meanings.

---

[24] kol po ser′vik al

[25] o va′re an

[26] o″vu la′shun, ov″u la′shun

[27] es′tro jen

[28] pro jes′tĕ rōn

[29] men″stroo a′shun

[30] kli mak′ter ik, kli″mak ter′ik

[31] men′o pawz

[32] men′sēz

[33] ah men″o re′ah

[34] dis″men or re′ah

[35] men″o ra′je ah

[36] me″tro ra′je ah, met″ro ra′je ah

WORD PARTS PERTAINING TO THE FEMALE REPRODUCTIVE SYSTEM

Word Part	Meaning
cervic/o	cervix (sometimes means the neck)
colp/o, vagin/o	vagina
gynec/o	female
hyster/o, uter/o	uterus
mamm/o, mast/o	breast
men/o	month
metr/o (occasionally metr/i)	uterine tissue (sometimes metr/o means measure)
oophor/o, ovar/o	ovary
salping/o	uterine tube (fallopian tube)
vulv/o	vulva

PROGRAMMED LEARNING

Practice using the word parts you have just learned. Remember to cover the answers in the left column and then to check each answer after you write it in the blank space.

cervical
vaginal
uterine
ovarian

1. Adjectives that pertain to the cervix, uterus, ovary, and vagina are written using combining forms that sound similar to the names of these structures. Use care with the endings and write words that mean
   pertaining to the cervix: _____
   pertaining to the vagina: _____
   pertaining to the uterus: _____
   pertaining to one or both ovaries: _____

vulval

2. Vulvar means pertaining to the vulva. Another word that means vulvar (its synonym) is _____.

colp/o

3. In addition to vagin/o, you learned another combining form that means vagina. Write that combining form: _____

vagina

colpocervicitis[37]

tissue

inside (or lining)

endometrium

uterus

hyster/o
uter/o

salping/o

salpingitis[40]

ovary

oophorectomy[42]

4. Colpo/cervical means pertaining to the cervix and the
   _____.

5. Use colpocervical as a model to write a word that means
   inflammation of the vagina and cervix:
   _____

6. The combining form metr/o means measurement or uterine
   _____. It is in this latter sense that metr/o will be
   used in the next two frames.

7. In what part of the uterus is the endometrium located?
   _____

8. Endometr/itis[38] is inflammation of the _____.

9. You have probably heard of a surgical procedure called a
   hysterectomy.[39] A hyster/ectomy is surgical removal of the
   _____.

10. Many medical words pertaining to the uterus use the combin-
    ing form that was presented in the last frame. Write two
    combining forms that mean the uterus: _____
    and _____

11. Uterine tubes carry ova from the ovary to the uterus. The com-
    bining form that means uterine tube is _____.

12. Inflammation of a uterine tube is _____.

13. Oophor/itis[41] is inflammation of an _____.

14. Write a term for surgical removal of an ovary:
    _____

---

[37] kol po ser vĭ si′tis   [40] sal″pin ji′tis
[38] en″do mĕ tri′tis   [41] o″of o ri′tis
[39] his″tĕ rek′to me   [42] o″of o rek′to me

gynec/o

15. Gynecology contains a combining form that means female. It is
    _____ .

gynecologist[43]

16. A physician who specializes in diseases of the female genital tract
    is a _____ .

men/o

17. Menstruation occurs at fairly regular intervals, approximately
    once each month. It is so named for this reason. The combining
    form that means month is _____ .

menstruation

18. Menses is another name for _____ . (Be careful
    with the spelling of this term, because it is frequently misspelled.)

menopause

19. Another name for the climacteric is formed by using men/o.
    This term is _____ .

menstruation

20. Metro/rrhagia means uterine bleeding occurring at a time other
    than during the menstrual period. Meno/rrhagia is excessive
    flow during _____ .

absence

21. The suffix -rrhea in amenorrhea means flow, or discharge.
    A/meno/rrhea means the _____ of menstrual
    flow when it is normally expected.

22. Use amenorrhea as a model to write a word that means painful
    menstruation (literal translation is difficult flow):

dysmenorrhea

_____

Terms Pertaining to Surgical Procedures of the Female Genitalia

colpoplasty[44] (colp/o, vagina, + -plasty, surgical repair): plastic surgery of the vagina
colporrhaphy[45] (-rrhaphy, suture): suture of the vagina

conization[46] of the cervix: excision of a cone of tissue from the cervix, performed to remove a lesion from the cervix or to obtain tissue for biopsy (this procedure is sometimes performed in conjunction with a D & C; see below)
dilation and curettage[47]: a surgical procedure that expands the cervical opening (dilation or dil-

[43] gi″ně kol′o jist, jin″ě kol′o jist
[44] kol′po plas″te
[45] kol por′ah fe

[46] co nǐ za′shun
[47] ku″rě tahzh′

atation) so that the uterine wall can be scraped (curettage); abbreviated D & C

hysterectomy (hyster/o, uterus): surgical removal of the uterus. Removal of the uterus through the abdominal wall is called an abdominal hysterectomy, or **laparohysterectomy**[48] (lapar/o, abdominal wall). Removal of the uterus through the vagina is called a **vaginal hysterectomy.**

laparoscopy[49] (lapar/o, abdominal wall, + -scopy, visually examining): abdominal exploration using a lighted instrument, the **laparoscope,**[50] which allows for direct visualization of the abdominal contents

laparotomy[51] (-tomy, incision): an abdominal operation; surgical opening of the abdomen done for various purposes

salpingectomy[52] (salping/o, uterine tube, + -ectomy, excision): surgical removal of a uterine tube

salpingo-oophorectomy[53] (oophor/o, ovary, + -ectomy, excision): removal of an ovary and its accompanying uterine tube. Bilateral salpingo-oophorectomy is removal of both ovaries and their uterine tubes.

salpingorrhaphy[54] (-rrhaphy, suture): suture of a uterine tube

tubal ligation[55]: surgical binding of the uterine tubes for elective sterilization (ligation means binding or tying).

EXERCISE I

Match the word parts in the left column with their meanings in the right column.

_____	1. colp/o	A.	abdominal wall
_____	2. hyster/o	B.	ovary
_____	3. lapar/o	C.	uterine tube
_____	4. oophor/o	D.	uterus
_____	5. salping/o	E.	vagina

(Check your answers with the solutions in the back of the book.)

EXERCISE II

Write letters in the blanks to correctly complete each word.

1. Surgical removal of the uterus is a __ __ __ __ __ __ectomy.
2. Plastic surgery of the vagina is __ __ __ __ __plasty.
3. Suture of the vagina is colpo __ __ __ __ __ __ __.
4. Removal of an ovary is __ __ __ __ __ __ectomy.
5. Suture of a uterine tube is __ __ __ __ __ __ __ __rrhaphy.
6. Tying or binding of a uterine tube for elective sterilization is a tubal __ __ __ __ __ __ __ __.

---

[48] lap″ah ro his″ter ek′to me
[49] lap″ah ros′ko pe
[50] lap′ah ro skōp
[51] lap ah rot′o me

[52] sal″pin jek′to me
[53] sal ping″go o″of o rek′to me
[54] sal″ping gor′ah fe
[55] too′bal li ga′shun

7. Use of a lighted instrument to allow for direct visualization of the abdominal contents is _ _ _ _ _ _scopy.
8. The surgical procedure that is abbreviated D & C is _ _ _ _ _ _ _ _ _ and

   _ _ _ _ _ _ _ _ _.
9. An abdominal incision is a _ _ _ _ _ _tomy.
10. Cervical _ _ _ _ _ _ _ _ _ _ _ is excision of a small cone of tissue from the cervix.
11. A vaginal _ _ _ _ _ _ _ _ is an instrument that is inserted into the vagina and used to examine the vagina and the cervix.
12. The study of diseases of the female reproductive organs is _ _ _ _ _ _logy.

(*Check your answers.*)

Diseases, Disorders, and Diagnostic Terms Pertaining to the Female Genitalia

cervical polyp[56]: a fibrous or mucous stalked tumor of the cervical mucosa (lining) (polyp is a general term for tumors that bleed easily and are found on mucous membranes)

colpitis[57] (colp/o, vagina, + -itis, inflammation): inflammation of the vagina; same as **vaginitis**[58]

colpocervicitis: inflammation of the vagina and cervix

colposcopy[59] (-scopy, visually examining): visual examination of vaginal and cervical tissue using a colposcope,[60] which magnifies the area to be examined

contraceptive[61] (contra-, against): any device, process, or method that prevents conception (pregnancy). **Oral contraceptives,** termed collo-quially "the pill," are chemicals that are similar to natural hormones and are taken by mouth.

endometriosis[62] (endo-, inside, + metr/i, uterine tissue, + -osis, condition): a condition in which tissue that somewhat resembles the endometrium is found abnormally in various locations in the pelvic cavity. (Endometriosis has an unusual spelling, so be careful.)

endometritis (-itis, inflammation): inflammation of the endometrium

fistula[63]: an abnormal, tubelike passage between two internal organs, or between an internal organ and the body surface. A **rectovaginal**[64] (rect/o, rectum) **fistula** is an abnormal opening between the rectum and the vagina. A **vesicovaginal**[65] (vesic/o, bladder) **fistula** is an abnormal opening between the bladder and the vagina.

hysteroptosis[66] (hyster/o, uterus, + -ptosis, sagging): prolapse of the uterus

oophoritis (oophor/o, ovary): an inflamed condition of an ovary

---

[56] pol′ip
[57] kol pi′tis
[58] vag″ĭ ni′tis
[59] kol pos′ko pe
[60] kol′po skōp
[61] kon″trah sep′tiv

[62] en″do me″tre o′sis
[63] fis′tu lah
[64] rek″to vaj′ĭ nal
[65] ves″i ko vag″ĭ nal
[66] his″ter op to′sis

oophorosalpingitis[67] (salping/o, uterine tube): inflammation of an ovary and its uterine tube

pelvic inflammatory disease: infection of the upper genital organs beyond the cervix, often involving the peritoneum and intestines (abbreviated PID)

salpingitis (salping/o, uterine tube): inflammation of a uterine tube

salpingocele[68] (-cele, hernia): hernial protrusion of a uterine tube

vulvitis[69] (vulv/o, vulva): inflammation of the vulva

EXERCISE III

Match terms in the right column with their meanings in the left column (not all selections will be used).

_____ 1. abnormal passage between two internal organs or between an internal organ and the body surface

_____ 2. device or method that prevents pregnancy

_____ 3. tumor occurring on a mucous membrane

A. contraceptive
B. fistula
C. polyp
D. prolapse

EXERCISE IV

Circle the correct answer to complete each sentence.

1. A word that means the same as vaginitis is (cervicitis, colpitis, salpingitis, vulvitis).
2. A condition in which tissue that somewhat resembles endometrium is found in an abnormal location in the pelvic cavity is called (endometritis, endometriosis, pelvic inflammatory disease, peritubal adhesions).
3. An examination using an instrument that magnifies the vaginal mucosa is called (colpitis, colposcopy, endometriosis, hysteroptosis).

---

[67] o of″o ro sal″pin ji′tis
[68] sal ping′go sel

[69] vul vi′tis

4. Prolapse of the uterus is (extrauterine, hysterectomy, hysteroptosis, intrauterine).
5. Inflammation of the inner lining of the uterus is (colpitis, endometritis, salpingitis, vulvitis).

(Check your answers.)

OBSTETRICS

Obstetrics[70] is the branch of medicine that specializes in the care of females during pregnancy and childbirth. The specialist is an **obstetrician.**[71] **Gestation,**[72] another word meaning pregnancy, is the period of time from conception to birth. **Parturition**[73] is a synonym for childbirth. **Antepartum**[74] (ante-, before) means before childbirth and **postpartum**[75] (post-, after) means after childbirth.

The combining form *par/o* is often used to form words referring to the bearing of offspring. A designation showing the number of pregnancies resulting in viable offspring is para I or para II (i.e., one or two pregnancies). Other designations are **unipara**[76] (uni-, one, + -para, female who has given birth), **bipara**[77] (bi-, two), and **tripara**[78] (tri-, three). **Nullipara**[79] (nulli-, none) refers to a woman who has never given birth to a viable offspring.

Fertilization of the egg by the sperm occurs most often in the uterine tube. The fertilized ovum (egg) usually implants in the endometrium. The **placenta** is the membrane through which the fetus derives nourishment during pregnancy. It is commonly called the *afterbirth* because it is expelled following delivery of the baby. A D & C might be performed to remove placental tissue that was not expelled.

In humans, the developing embryo is called a **fetus** after 8 weeks. **Fetal**[80] (fet/o, fetus) is an adjective that refers to the fetus. Within a few days after fertilization has occurred a hormone called human chorionic gonadotropin (HCG) is produced, and this can be detected in body fluids. Testing for this hormone in urine or blood can indicate if a female is pregnant. HCG can be detected long before other signs of pregnancy appear.

Ultrasonography[81] (ultra-, beyond, + son/o, sound, + -graphy,

---

[70] ob stet′riks
[71] ob″stĕ trish′un
[72] jes ta′shun
[73] par″tu rish′un
[74] an″te par′tum
[75] pōst par′tum

[76] u nip′ah rah
[77] bip′ah rah
[78] trip′ah rah
[79] nuh lip′ah rah
[80] fe′tal
[81] ul″trah son og′rah fe

recording), also called **ultrasound,**[82] provides an image of the developing fetus. It is used to obtain images of organs and tissues throughout the body for diagnostic and therapeutic purposes. Ultrasonography has many uses in obstetrics, including the detection of an embryo that has implanted outside the uterus. Such abnormal implantation is called an **extrauterine** or **ectopic**[83] **pregnancy.** The word *ectopic,* derived from ecto- (outside) and top/o (location), means located outside the usual place.

Prenatal[84] (nat/i, birth) and **postnatal**[85] mean happening before birth and after birth, respectively. A **neonate**[86] (ne/o, new) is a newborn infant up to 6 weeks of age, and this period of time is known as the **neonatal**[87] period.

Several word parts you need to remember are presented in the following list. **Memorize** the meanings of all word parts shown.

WORD PARTS RELATED TO OBSTETRIC TERMS

Word Part	Meaning
amni/o	amnion (fetal membrane)
fet/o	fetus
nat/i	birth
par/o	to bear offspring
-para	a female who has given birth

ADDITIONAL WORD PARTS

Word Part	Meaning
extra-	outside
gon/o	genitals or reproduction
lapar/o	abdominal wall
rect/o	rectum
son/o	sound

---

[82] ul'trah sownd
[83] ek top'ik
[84] pre na'tal

[85] pōst na'tal
[86] ne'o nāt
[87] ne"o na'tal

ADDITIONAL WORD PARTS (Continued)

Word Part	Meaning
tox/o	poison
tri-	three
ultra-	beyond or excess
vesic/o	bladder

EXERCISE V

Write the meaning of each underlined word part in the blank spaces.

1. neo<u>nat</u>al _____
2. <u>tri</u>para _____
3. <u>nulli</u>para _____
4. <u>ultra</u>sound _____
5. uni<u>para</u> _____
6. ultra<u>sono</u>graphy _____

EXERCISE VI

Match the terms in the left column with their meanings in the right column.

_____ 1. antepartum   A. pregnancy
_____ 2. gestation   B. childbirth
_____ 3. parturition   C. before birth
_____ 4. postpartum   D. after birth

EXERCISE VII

Write letters in the blanks to complete each word correctly.

1. A woman who has had one child is a unipara. A __ __para has produced two children.
2. A developing embryo is called a __ __ __ __ __ after 8 weeks.
3. Abnormal implantation of a fertilized ovum outside the uterus is called an ec __ __ __ __ __ pregnancy.
4. A term that means after childbirth is __ __ __ __natal.
5. The first 6 weeks after a child is born is the __ __ __natal period.

(Check your answers.)

Additional Terms Related to Obstetrics

amnion[88]: the innermost of the membranes that surround the developing fetus. This transparent sac, also called the **amniotic**[89] **sac,** holds the fetus suspended in amniotic fluid.

amniocentesis[90] (amni/o, amnion, + -centesis, puncture): puncture of the amniotic sac through the abdomen to remove amniotic fluid. The material that is removed can be studied to detect genetic disorders or other abnormalities.

amniotomy[91] (-tomy, incision): surgical rupture of the fetal membranes, performed to induce or expedite labor

cesarean[92] **section:** incision through the walls of the abdomen and uterus for delivery of a fetus (abbreviated as C section)

Down's syndrome: a congenital condition characterized by mild to severe mental retardation and caused by an abnormality, usually the presence of three chromosome #21, rather than the expected pair (this condition is, less desirably, also called mongolism)

fetal monitoring (fet/o, fetus): assessment of the fetus in utero, usually with respect to its heartbeat (by electrocardiography)

EXERCISE VIII   *Circle the correct answer to complete each sentence.*

1. The transparent sac that encloses the fetus in utero is called the (amniocentesis, amniotic, congenital, trisomic) sac.
2. A congenital condition of the newborn marked by mental retardation is (Down's syndrome, cesarean section, ectopic pregnancy, jaundice).
3. Surgical rupture of the fetal membrane is (amniocentesis, amniotomy, cesarean section, fetal monitoring).
4. Surgical puncture of the amnion is (amniotic, amniocentesis, amniotomy, cesarean section).
5. The membrane through which the fetus receives nourishment is the (fistula, HCG, ovary, placenta).

(Check your answers.)

MALE GENITALIA   Male reproductive organs include the **testes** or **testicles,** which produce sperm, a number of **ducts** for transporting the sperm, several **glands** that produce fluid, and the **penis**[93] (Fig. 10–2).

The **scrotum**[94] is a pouch of loose skin that contains the two testes and their accessory organs (the singular form of testes is testis). The testes produce sperm and a hormone responsible for the development

---

[88] am′ne on
[89] an″ne ot′ik
[90] am″ne o sen te′sis
[91] am″ne ot′o me

[92] se sa′re an
[93] pe′nis
[94] skro′tum

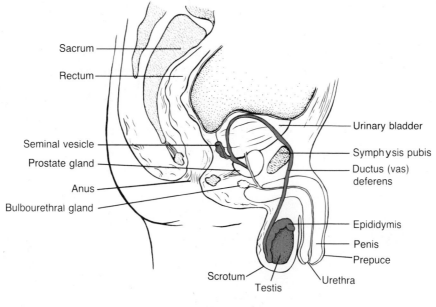

FIGURE 10-2

Male genitalia *(cross section)*. The urinary bladder, rectum, and anus are not structures of the reproductive system but are labeled to show their positions relative to reproductive structures. (From Leonard, P.C.: *Building a Medical Vocabulary*. 2nd ed. Philadelphia, W.B. Saunders, 1988.)

and maintenance of male secondary sex characteristics, **testosterone.**[95] An important duct, the **ductus deferens** (also called the vas deferens), transports sperm from the testes to the urethra, where they are discharged.

Sperm leave the male's body in **semen,**[96] the fluid that is discharged from the penis at the height of sexual excitement. Seminal vesicles[97] (semin/o, seed or semen) serve as a reservoir for semen until it is discharged. (As you previously learned in this chapter, vesic/o means bladder. The term *vesicle*, however, means a small sac or bladder containing fluid, or a small blisterlike elevation on the skin containing serous fluid. Seminal vesicles refer to small sacs that store semen, whereas vesicular rash refers to an eruption of blisters on the skin.) The **seminal vesicles,** the **prostate,**[98] and other **glands** produce

---

[95] tes tos'tĕ rōn

[96] se'men

[97] sem'ĭ nal ves'ĭ kalz

[98] pros'tāt

fluids necessary for survival of the sperm. The prostate is also called the prostate gland.

Spermatogenesis[99] (spermat/o, sperm, + -genesis, producing or originating) is production of sperm. Sperm is short for **spermatozoa**, the mature male sex cells. **Spermatocidal**[100] (spermat/o, sperm, + -cidal, killing) pertains to the killing of sperm. Contraceptive foams and creams are spermatocidal, and as such are designed to prevent pregnancy.

Several important word parts pertain to male reproductive organs. Commit the meaning of the following word parts to **memory.**

WORD PARTS PERTAINING TO MALE REPRODUCTIVE ORGANS

Word Part	Meaning
orchi/o, orchid/o, test/o, testic/o	testes
pen/o*	penis
prostat/o	prostate
scrot/o	scrotum, bag
semin/o	semen
spermat/o	sperm
urethr/o	urethra
vas/o	vessel or duct—sometimes ductus (vas) deferens

* In some words, pen/o means punishment (e.g., penology is the study of punishment).

Terms Pertaining to Surgical Procedures of the Male Genitalia

circumcision[101]: surgical removal of the end of the foreskin that covers the head of the penis. This is usually performed shortly after birth for hygienic reasons.

orchidectomy[102] (orchid/o, testes, + -ectomy, excision): surgical removal of a testicle (often done to treat malignancy of a testicle). Excision of both testes is **castration.**[103] **Orchiectomy**[104] is a synonym for orchidectomy.

orchidoplasty[105] (-plasty, surgical repair): plastic surgery of the testis, particularly the surgery

---

[99] sper″mah to jen′e sis
[100] sper″mah to si′dal
[101] ser″kum sizh′un
[102] or″kĭ dek′to me

[103] kas tra′shun
[104] or″ke ek′to me
[105] or′kĭ do plas″te

performed to correct a testicle that has not descended properly into the scrotum

orchiopexy[106] (-pexy, surgical fixation): surgical fixation of an undescended testicle in the scrotum

prostatectomy[107] (prostat/o, prostate, + -ectomy, excision): removal of all or part of the prostate

transurethral[108] **prostatectomy** (trans-, across, + urethr/o, urethra): removal of part of the prostate gland through an incision in the urethral wall (abbreviated as TURP). It is also called **transurethral resection,** or TUR. Resection[109] is a term that means partial excision of a structure.

vasectomy[110] (vas/o, vas deferens, + -ectomy,

excision): removal of all or a segment of the vas deferens (usually done bilaterally to produce sterility)

vasoplasty[111] (-plasty, surgical repair): surgical repair of the vas deferens, done to correct a defect of the vas deferens or to reverse the effects of a vasectomy

vasorrhaphy[112] (-rrhaphy, suture): surgical suture of the vas deferens

vasostomy[113] (-stomy, new opening): formation of an opening into the ductus deferens; has sometimes been successful in reversing the effect of a vasectomy

---

EXERCISE IX

Match the word parts in the left column with their meanings in the right column (not all answers will be used, and some answers will be used more than once).

_____ 1. orchi/o
_____ 2. orchid/o
_____ 3. test/o
_____ 4. urethr/o
_____ 5. vas/o

A. ductus deferens
B. penis
C. prostate
D. scrotum
E. testes
F. ureter
G. urethra

EXERCISE X

The following are adjectives that pertain to various aspects of male reproduction. Write the name of the structure or aspect to which each adjective refers.

1. seminal _____
2. scrotal _____
3. penile _____
4. prostatic _____
5. testicular _____

---

[106] or"ke o pek'se
[107] pros"tah tek'to me
[108] trans"u re'thral
[109] re sek'shun

[110] vah sek'to me
[111] vas'o plas"te
[112] vas or'ah fe
[113] vah sos'to me

EXERCISE XI

Using word parts you have learned, write letters in the blanks to correctly complete each sentence.

1. An important male hormone produced by the testes is __ __ __ __ __sterone.
2. The term for surgical fixation of an undescended testicle is __ __ __ __ __opexy.
3. Surgical removal of the end of the foreskin that covers the head of the penis is __ __ __ __ __ __cision.
4. Surgical suture of the ductus deferens is __ __ __ __rrhaphy.
5. Surgical removal of a segment of the ductus deferens is a vas __ __ __ __ __ __.
6. Surgical removal of a testicle is __ __ __ __ __ __ectomy.
7. Surgical removal of all or part of the prostate is called a __ __ __ __ __ __ __ectomy.

(Check your answers.)

Diseases, Disorders, and Diagnostic Terms Pertaining to the Male Genitalia

cryptorchidism[114] (crypt/o, hidden, + orchid/o, testis, + -ism, condition): undescended testicles; failure of the testicles to descend into the scrotum before birth

hydrocele[115] (hydr/o, water, + -cele, hernia): accumulation of fluid in a saclike cavity, especially serous tumors of the testes or associated parts. Serous (ser/o, serum, + -ous, pertaining to) means like serum or producing or containing serum.

orchiditis[116] or **orchitis**[117] (orchid/o or orchi/o, testis, + -itis, inflammation): inflammation of a testis. (Notice the spelling of *orchitis*. In joining orchi/o + -itis, one *i* is dropped so no double *i* appears in the word.)

prostatic hypertrophy[118] (hyper-, excessive, + -trophy, nutrition): enlargement of the prostate. Hypertrophy means an increase in the size of an organ or structure by enlargement of the existing cells, rather than an increase in the number of cells. Prostatic hypertrophy usually results in urethral obstruction and interferes with urination. This condition is generally benign (not malignant). **Benign prostatic hypertrophy** is abbreviated as BPH.

prostatitis[119] (-itis, inflammation): inflammation of the prostate

EXERCISE XII

Using word parts you have learned, write letters in the blanks to correctly complete each sentence.

1. Crypt __ __ __ __ __ __ __ __ __ means undescended testicles.

---

[114] krip tor'ki dizm
[115] hi'dro sēl
[116] or"ki di'tis
[117] or ki'tis
[118] pros tat'ik hi per'tro fe
[119] pros"tah ti'tis

2. Enlargement of the prostate is __ __ __ __ __ __ __ __ __ hypertrophy.

3. The term that means inflammation of the prostate is __ __ __ __ __ __ __ __ __ __ __.

4. A synonym for orchiditis is __ __ __ __ __ __ __ __.

5. A term that means an increase in the size of an organ or structure by enlargement of existing cells is __ __ __ __ __trophy.

6. BPH is an abbreviation for __ __ __ __ __ __ prostatic hypertrophy.

(Check your answers.)

SEXUALLY TRANSMITTED DISEASES

A disease acquired through sexual contact is a **sexually transmitted disease** (STD), formerly called venereal disease (*venereal* was named for Venus, goddess of love). Generally, sexually transmitted diseases cause one of the following problems: male urethritis (urethr/o, urethra, + -itis, inflammation), female lower genitourinary tract infection, and vaginitis (vagin/o, vagina). **Genitourinary**[120] pertains to the genitals (genit/o) and the urinary organs (ur/o, urine or urinary tract).

Gonorrhea[121] is a contagious genitourinary infection caused by the bacterium that is commonly called the **gonococcus.**[122] Both terms use the word part gon/o, which means reproduction or the genitals. You learned earlier that -rrhea means flow or discharge. In gonorrhea, -rrhea refers to the heavy discharge that often appears as a symptom in this disease. Gonorrhea is caused by the gonococcus. A coccus (pl., cocci) is a spherical bacteria.

Syphilis[123] is another STD caused by the bacteria that are commonly called **spirochetes.**[124] (In spirochete spir/o means spiral, but sometimes spir/o is used to mean to breathe in terms such as *spirometer*, which is an apparatus that measures the volume of air inhaled and exhaled. The -chete in spirochete means hair, referring to the thin hairlike appearance of the organism, but the important thing to remember is that one type of spirochete causes syphilis.) Another important term is **chancre,**[125] the primary lesion that appears 2 to 3 weeks after a person is infected with syphilis.

Herpes genitalis,[126] or **genital herpes,** is a highly infectious STD characterized by blisters on the genital organs. Unlike gonorrhea and syphilis, genital herpes is caused by a virus, and is more difficult to

---

[120] jen″ĭ to u′rĭ ner e
[121] gon″o re′ah
[122] gon″o kok′us
[123] sif′ĭ lis

[124] spi′ro kētz
[125] shang′ker
[126] her′pēz jen ĭ tal′is

treat. The term *herpes* as a single word, however, is imprecise; at one time it was used to indicate eruptions caused by a virus, especially the virus that causes cold sores or fever blisters.

Acquired immune deficiency syndrome (AIDS), another viral infection, is an epidemic and usually fatal form of immunodeficiency. **Immunodeficiency**[127] (immun/o, immune) means a lowered or deficient immune response. A **syndrome**[128] is a condition with a defined set of signs and symptoms that are not necessarily caused by the same disease. (The terms *syndrome* and *disease* are often used indiscriminately.) AIDS is characterized by opportunistic infections and malignant disease, with no known cause for the immunodeficiency. The term *malignant* implies that the condition tends to become progressively worse. Cancerous growths are called **malignancies**.[129] Opportunistic infections occur because of the weakened state of the host. AIDS is not only transmitted through sexual intercourse but also through contaminated needles, blood, blood products, and other body fluids of the infected person.

No attempt is made to discuss all sexually transmitted diseases in this chapter. You might want to consult other sources for additional information concerning STDs.

EXERCISE XIII

Match the terms in the left column with the clues in the right column.

_____ 1. chancre
_____ 2. immunodefi-
            ciency
_____ 3. gonococcus
_____ 4. spirochete

A. characteristic of AIDS
B. primary lesion of syphilis
C. causative agent of syphilis
D. causative agent of gonorrhea

EXERCISE XIV

Using word parts you have learned, write letters in the blank spaces to correctly complete each sentence.

1. Another name for venereal disease is
   __ __ __ __ __ __ __ __ transmitted disease.
2. AIDS is an abbreviation for acquired __ __ __ __ __ __ deficiency syndrome.
3. An infection that occurs because of the opportunity afforded

---

[127] im″u no dĕ fish′en se
[128] sin′drōm

[129] mah lig′nan sēz

by the weakened physiologic state of the host is an

— — — — — — — — — — — — — — — infection.

4. The microorganism that causes gonorrhea is commonly called the gono — — — — — — —.

5. A term sometimes used instead of *disease* but that actually means a condition having a collection of signs and symptoms that are not necessarily caused by the same disease is

— — — — — — — —.

6. One type of sexually transmitted disease is gono-

— — — — —.

7. Another type of sexually transmitted disease is

s — — — — — — —.

(Check your answers.)

Several word parts have been introduced in this chapter that do not refer specifically to the reproductive system, and are also found in other terms. Be sure that you **know the meaning** of these word parts, which are listed below.

ADDITIONAL WORD PARTS

Word Part	Meaning
-cidal	killing
genit/o	genitals
hydr/o	water
immun/o	immune
ser/o	serum
spir/o	spiral, or to breathe
trans-	across
ur/o	urine or urinary tract

Comprehensive Review Exercises

WORK THE FOLLOWING EXERCISES TO TEST YOUR UNDERSTANDING OF THE MATERIAL IN CHAPTER 10. IT IS BEST TO DO ALL THE REVIEW EXERCISES BEFORE CHECKING YOUR ANSWERS.

A. Write the meaning of each underlined word part in the blank spaces.

1. <u>gon</u>ads _____

2. <u>gyneco</u>logy _____

3. <u>cervic</u>al _____ or _____

4. endo<u>metr</u>ium _____

5. <u>men</u>struation _____

6. <u>sero</u>us _____

7. <u>urethr</u>itis _____

8. spermato<u>cid</u>al _____

9. pre<u>nat</u>al _____

10. ultra<u>son</u>ography _____

11. <u>immuno</u>deficiency _____

12. <u>tri</u>para _____

13. <u>pen</u>ile _____

14. <u>hydro</u>cele _____

B. Match the word parts in the left column with their meanings in the right column.

_____ 1. colp/o   A. abdominal wall

_____ 2. hyster/o   B. breast

_____ 3. lapar/o   C. ductus deferens

_____ 4. mamm/o   D. ovary

_____ 5. oophor/o   E. testis

_____ 6. orchi/o   F. uterine tube

_____ 7. salping/o   G. uterus

_____ 8. vas/o   H. vagina

C. Using word parts you have learned, write letters in the blanks to correctly complete each sentence.

1. The tissue that forms the lining of the uterus is endo-
   __ __ __ __ __.

2. Pertaining to the vagina and cervix is __ __ __ __ __cervical.

3. Menstruation is also called __ __ __ __ __ __.

4. Inflammation of a uterine tube is __ __ __ __ __ __ __itis.

5. Surgical removal of an ovary is __ __ __ __ __ __ectomy.

6. Another term for vaginitis is ＿ ＿ ＿ ＿itis.

7. Any device that prevents pregnancy is a
   ＿ ＿ ＿ ＿ ＿ ＿ceptive.

8. Another name for pregnancy is ＿ ＿ ＿ ＿ ＿tion.

9. Production of sperm is ＿ ＿ ＿ ＿ ＿ ＿ ＿ ＿genesis.

10. Surgical removal of a testicle is ＿ ＿ ＿ ＿ ＿ ＿ectomy.

11. An undescended testicle is ＿ ＿ ＿ ＿ ＿orchidism.

12. Excision of all or part of the prostate is

    ＿ ＿ ＿ ＿ ＿ ＿ ＿ ＿ ＿ ＿ ＿ ＿ ＿.

D. Circle the correct answer to complete each sentence.

1. The reproductive organs are called the (genitalia, gonadotropin, uteri, vulva).

2. Which of the following means within the uterus? (cervix uteri, extrauterine, intrauterine, myometrium)

3. Removal of an ovary and its accompanying uterine tube is a(n) (abdominal hysterectomy, vaginal hysterectomy, salpingo-oophorectomy, tubal ligation).

4. Menopause is also called (amenorrhea, climacteric, dysmenorrhea, fistula).

5. Inflammation of the inner lining of the uterus is (cervicitis, endometriosis, endometritis, vaginitis).

6. A surgical procedure that expands the cervical opening so that the uterine wall can be scraped is called (conization of the cervix, dilation and curettage, hysterectomy, laparoscopy).

7. Vaginal is (a noun that means the birth canal, an adjective that refers to the birth canal, a noun that means the womb, an adjective that refers to the womb).

8. An abnormal tubelike passage is a(n) (adhesion, colposcopy, fistula, polyp).

9. Prolapse of the uterus is (endometriosis, endometritis, hysteroptosis, salpingocele).

10. An inflammation of the external female genital structure is (colpitis, urethrovaginitis, vaginitis, vulvitis).

11. Childbirth is (gestation, neonatality, obstetrics, parturition).

12. Abnormal implantation of an embryo outside the uterus is a(n) (ectopic, intrauterine, prenatal, postnatal) pregnancy.

13. A tumor found on a mucous membrane is a(n) (curettage, ovum, Pap, polyp).

14. Surgical rupture of the fetal membranes is (amnion, amniotomy, colporrhaphy, cesarean section).

15. The study of diseases of the female reproductive organs is (gynecology, obstetrics, orchidism, penology).

16. Which of the following abbreviations means a test for early diagnosis of cancer of the uterus? (Pap, PID, TUR, TURP)

17. Excessive flow during menstruation is (dysmenorrhea, menorrhagia, menses, metrorrhagia).

18. Surgical removal of the end of the foreskin is (castration, circumcision, episiotomy, orchiectomy).

19. A word that means after childbirth is (antepartum, bipara, postpartum, unipara).

20. A hormone important in the development and maintenance of male sexual characteristics is (estrogen, chorionic gonadotropin, progesterone, testosterone).

21. Which of the following provides an image of the developing fetus? (amniocentesis, colposcopy, laparoscopy, ultrasonography)

22. Removal of all or a section of the ductus deferens is (orchidoplasty, orchiopexy, vasectomy, vasoplasty).

23. A serous tumor of the testis is called a(n) (hydrocele, metastasis, orchitis, phimosis).

24. Which of the following is a characteristic of early syphilis? (chancre, gonococcus, heavy discharge, immunodeficiency)

25. An STD characterized by blisters on the genital organs is (AIDS, gonorrhea, herpes genitalis, male urethritis).

E. Write the word for which each meaning is given:

1. developing human in utero after 8 weeks _____

2. pertaining to the ovaries _____

3. inflammation of the vagina and cervix _____

4. surgical removal of the uterus _____

5. inflammation of an ovary _____

6. absence of menstrual flow (when normally expected)

   _____

7. plastic surgery of the vagina _____

8. surgical opening of the abdomen _____

9. excision of a uterine tube _____

10. newborn infant _____

Review

11

Review of Chapters 1 to 10

OBJECTIVES

> **After completing the material in *Quick and Easy Medical Terminology* you will be able to**
>
> 1. Recognize and write the meaning of prefixes, suffixes, and combining forms that were presented in the chapter material.
> 2. Write the correct word part when presented with its meaning.
> 3. Analyze medical terms presented in the material and select the correct response from several answers.
> 4. Write the correct medical term when presented with its meaning or description.
> 5. Demonstrate understanding of the rules for using word parts by combining them correctly to write medical terms.

OUTLINE

SELF-TESTING
I. Writing the meaning of word parts
II. Writing word parts
III. Answering multiple-choice questions
IV. Writing medical terms

SELF-TESTING

This chapter is included to enable you to test yourself on how well you remember the material. Work all questions in this review if you completed all chapters in the book. Each question is presented with its relevant chapter number. If you did not complete all chapters in the book, eliminate the questions relating to chapters that were not covered.

Four types of questions are included:

    I. Writing the meaning of prefixes, suffixes, and combining forms

    II. Writing word parts

    III. Answering multiple-choice questions

    IV. Writing medical terms

It is better to do all questions in a set before checking the answers. Grade your answers as though it were an actual test. Make a special study sheet for yourself and list all word parts and their meanings that you missed in the first two sets.

Look through the chapter material and find the correct answer for all multiple-choice questions that you missed. Then look at the answer that you originally selected and determine why it is incorrect.

Carefully look at how words are spelled when you check the medical terms that you wrote in the fourth set of questions. Also, make a list of all word parts that you could not remember or that you wrote incorrectly.

Refer to your study sheet several times before taking the test that your instructor prepares. If time permits, read all chapters again. The following review is a representative sample of chapter material but does not include every term.

I. Writing the Meaning of Word Parts

Write the meaning of each word part that is listed.

Word Part	Meaning	Chapter Reference
1. a-	_____	3
2. acr/o	_____	4
3. aden/o	_____	2
4. aer/o	_____	3
5. alb/o	_____	3
6. -algia	_____	2
7. amyl/o	_____	2
8. an-	_____	3

Word Part	Meaning	Chapter Reference
9. angi/o	_____	2
10. ante-	_____	3
11. anti-	_____	3
12. arthr/o	_____	5
13. -ase	_____	2
14. atel/o	_____	7
15. ather/o	_____	6
16. bi-	_____	3
17. blast/o	_____	3
18. blephar/o	_____	2
19. brady-	_____	3
20. carcin/o	_____	3
21. cardi/o	_____	2
22. carp/o	_____	5
23. caud/o	_____	4
24. -cele	_____	2
25. -centesis	_____	2
26. cephal/o	_____	3
27. cerebr/o	_____	2
28. cervic/o	_____	5, 10
29. cheil/o	_____	8
30. chir/o	_____	2
31. chlor/o	_____	3
32. cholecyst/o	_____	4, 8
33. chondr/o	_____	5
34. -cidal	_____	10
35. clavicul/o	_____	5
36. colp/o	_____	10
37. coni/o	_____	7
38. contra-	_____	3
39. cost/o	_____	5

Word Part	Meaning	Chapter Reference
40. crin/o	_____	4
41. cry/o	_____	3
42. crypt/o	_____	3
43. cutane/o	_____	2
44. cyan/o	_____	3
45. cyst/o	_____	4, 9
46. -cyte	_____	3
47. dacry/o	_____	4
48. dactyl/o	_____	4
49. de-	_____	5, 8
50. dent/o	_____	8
51. dermat/o	_____	2
52. dia-	_____	3
53. dips/o	_____	3
54. dist/o	_____	4
55. dors/o	_____	4
56. dys-	_____	3
57. ech/o	_____	6
58. -ectasis	_____	2
59. ecto-	_____	3
60. -emesis	_____	2
61. -emia	_____	4, 6, 8, 9
62. en-	_____	3
63. encephal/o	_____	2
64. endo-	_____	3
65. enter/o	_____	8
66. epi-	_____	3
67. erythr/o	_____	3
68. esthesi/o	_____	3
69. eu-	_____	3
70. ex-	_____	3

Word Part	Meaning	Chapter Reference
71. extra-	_____	6, 10
72. gastr/o	_____	8
73. gen/o	_____	3
74. geront/o	_____	3
75. gingiv/o	_____	8
76. gloss/o	_____	8
77. glyc/o	_____	2
78. gon/o	_____	10
79. -gram	_____	3
80. -graph	_____	3
81. -graphy	_____	3
82. gynec/o	_____	10
83. hemat/o	_____	4, 9
84. hemi-	_____	3
85. hepat/o	_____	4, 8
86. hidr/o	_____	4
87. hist/o	_____	3
88. home/o	_____	6, 7
89. hydr/o	_____	4, 10
90. hyper-	_____	2
91. hypo-	_____	3
92. hyster/o	_____	4, 10
93. -iasis	_____	2
94. -ic	_____	2
95. in-	_____	3
96. infer/o	_____	4
97. inter-	_____	3
98. intra-	_____	3
99. -ism	_____	2
100. -ist	_____	2
101. -itis	_____	2

Word Part	Meaning	Chapter Reference
102. -ium	_____	2
103. kinesi/o	_____	3
104. lacrim/o	_____	4
105. lact/o	_____	2
106. lapar/o	_____	4, 10
107. -lepsy	_____	3
108. leuk/o	_____	3
109. lingu/o	_____	8
110. lip/o	_____	2
111. lith/o	_____	2
112. -logist	_____	2
113. -logy	_____	3
114. -lysin	_____	3
115. -lysis	_____	2
116. -lytic	_____	3
117. odont/o	_____	8
118. optic/o	_____	3
119. orchi/o	_____	10
120. -osis	_____	2
121. -ous	_____	2
122. para-	_____	3
123. -para	_____	10
124. -pathy	_____	2
125. -phagy	_____	3
126. phren/o	_____	7
127. post-	_____	3
128. pneum/o	_____	7
129. pre-	_____	3
130. primi-	_____	3
131. proct/o	_____	8
132. proxim/o	_____	4

Word Part	Meaning	Chapter Reference
133. psych/o	_____	3
134. pulm/o	_____	7
135. rachi/o	_____	5
136. radi/o	_____	5, 6
137. retro-	_____	3
138. schiz/o	_____	3
139. semi-	_____	3
140. somat/o	_____	4
141. son/o	_____	6, 9, 10
142. spir/o	_____	7, 10
143. sub-	_____	3
144. supra-	_____	3
145. tetra-	_____	3
146. thromb/o	_____	6
147. ultra-	_____	10
148. uni-	_____	3
149. vas/o	_____	2
150. -y	_____	2

II. Writing Word Parts

Write the word part(s) indicated for each of the following (p, prefix; s, suffix; cf, combining form). For example, for an extremity (cf), you would write the combining form *acr/o* in the blank space.

Meaning	Word Part	Chapter Reference
1. bile (cf)	_____	
	or _____	8
2. wrist (cf)	_____	5
3. coccyx (cf)	_____	5
4. large intestine (cf)	_____	4, 8
5. skull (cf)	_____	5
6. surgical removal (s)	_____	2

Meaning	Word Part	Chapter Reference
7. swelling (s)	_____	2
8. thigh bone (cf)	_____	5
9. fiber (cf)	_____	3
10. voice box (cf)	_____	7
11. toward the side (cf)	_____	4
12. lymph or lymphatics (cf)	_____	4, 6
13. large or enlarged (s)	_____	2
14. bad (p)	_____	
	or _____	3
15. softening (s)	_____	2
16. breast (cf)	_____	
	or _____	2
17. excessive preoccupation (s)	_____	2
18. middle (p, cf)	_____	
	and _____	3, 4
19. large (p)	_____	3
20. black (cf)	_____	3
21. month (cf)	_____	10
22. measure or uterine tissue (cf)	_____	3
23. instrument used to measure (s)	_____	3
24. process of measuring (s)	_____	3
25. small (p)	_____	3
26. first (p)	_____	3
27. many (p)	_____	
	or _____	3
28. muscle (cf)	_____	
	or _____	5, 6
29. fungus (cf)	_____	3

Meaning	Word Part	Chapter Reference
30. bone marrow or spinal cord (cf)	_____	5, 6
31. sleep (cf)	_____	3
32. nose (cf)	_____	
	or _____	7
33. new (cf)	_____	3
34. dead or death (cf)	_____	3
35. kidney (cf)	_____	
	or _____	9
36. nerve (cf)	_____	2
37. none (p)	_____	3
38. resembling (s)	_____	2
39. little (s)	_____	7
40. tumor (s, cf)	_____	
	and _____	2, 3
41. umbilicus (cf)	_____	4
42. nail (cf)	_____	4
43. ovary (cf)	_____	
	or _____	10
44. eye (cf)	_____	2
45. mouth (cf)	_____	
	or _____	8
46. appetite (s)	_____	8
47. straight (cf)	_____	3
48. sugar (s)	_____	2
49. bone (cf)	_____	2
50. ear (cf)	_____	2
51. oxygen (cf)	_____	7
52. pancreas (cf)	_____	8
53. kneecap (cf)	_____	5
54. disease (cf)	_____	3
55. deficiency (s)	_____	2

Meaning	Word Part	Chapter Reference
56. digestion (s)	_____	8
57. around (p)	_____	3
58. surgical fixation (s)	_____	2
59. drugs or medicine (cf)	_____	3
60. speech (cf)	_____	3
61. vein (cf)	_____	
	or _____	6
62. abnormal fear (s)	_____	2
63. voice (cf)	_____	3
64. light (cf)	_____	3
65. surgical repair (s)	_____	2
66. paralysis (s)	_____	3
67. breathing (s)	_____	7
68. prolapse (s)	_____	2
69. pus (cf)	_____	3
70. renal pelvis (cf)	_____	9
71. fire (cf)	_____	2
72. hemorrhage (s)	_____	
	or _____	2
73. suture (s)	_____	2
74. flow or discharge (s)	_____	2
75. rupture (s)	_____	2
76. uterine tube (cf)	_____	10
77. hard or hardening (s)	_____	3
78. instrument used for viewing (s)	_____	3
79. process of visually examining (s)	_____	2
80. semen (cf)	_____	10
81. saliva or salivary gland (cf)	_____	4, 8
82. cramp or twitching (s)	_____	2

	Meaning	Word Part	Chapter Reference
83.	sperm (cf)	_____	10
84.	uterus (cf)	_____	
		or _____	10
85.	vertebra (cf)	_____	
		or _____	5
86.	stopping or controlling (s)	_____	2
87.	breastbone (cf)	_____	5
88.	formation of an opening (s)	_____	2
89.	fast (p)	_____	3
90.	heat (cf)	_____	3
91.	chest (cf)	_____	4, 5, 7
92.	instrument used for cutting (s)	_____	2
93.	incision (s)	_____	2
94.	place, position (cf)	_____	3
95.	poison (cf)	_____	10
96.	windpipe (cf)	_____	7
97.	across (p)	_____	10
98.	three (p)	_____	3
99.	surgical crushing (s)	_____	2
100.	nutrition (cf)	_____	3
101.	urine or urinary tract (cf)	_____	4, 8, 9, 10
102.	vagina (cf)	_____	
		or _____	10
103.	vagus nerve (cf)	_____	8
104.	ductus deferens (cf)	_____	2
105.	belly side (cf)	_____	4
106.	yellow (cf)	_____	3

III. Multiple-Choice Questions

Circle the correct answer to complete each sentence.

Chapter 2

1. The suffix -centesis means (excision, incision, surgical puncture, surgical fixation).
2. The suffix -malacia means (abnormal fear, abnormal softening, hemorrhage, pain).
3. Which of the following means vomiting? (emesis, malacia, stasis, spasm)
4. Which of the following means breaking down or digestion of proteins? (protease, proteinase, proteogenesis, proteolysis)
5. Pertaining to the ear is (dermal, neuralgia, ophthalmic, otic).
6. Which of the following means examining the colon? (colectasis, colopexy, coloscopy, colostomy)
7. Mastitis is (excision, inflammation, sagging, surgical fixation) of the breast.
8. Excision of a small piece of living tissue for microscopic examination is called a(n) (adenectomy, biopsy, plastic surgery, ptosis).
9. Suture of a blood vessel is (angiectomy, angioplasty, angiorrhaphy, angiorrhexis).
10. Gastrocele is (any disease, enlargement, herniation, stretching) of the stomach.

Chapter 3

11. Within a cell is (extracellular, intercellular, intracellular, multicellular).
12. Normal thyroid activity is (euthyroidism, hypothyroidism, hyperthyroidism, parathyroidism).
13. Any condition that renders a particular line of treatment undesirable is a(n) (anticonvulsive, antacid, contraindication, malabsorption).
14. A weak voice is (dysphagia, dysphonia, dystrophic, dystrophy).
15. Which of the following words does *not* pertain to vision? (myopia, oncologist, optician, optometrist)
16. Excessive thirst is (exogenous, hyperthermia, neoplasm, polydipsia).
17. Death of tissue is (diathermy, epilepsy, necrosis, pyoderma).
18. Absence of speech is (aphasia, aphonia, ectopic, hemiplegia).
19. Which of the following terms does *not* contain a prefix that indicates location? (mesonasal, postnasal, supratonsillar, tachykinesia)
20. Sudden attacks of sleep occurring at intervals is called (bradyphasia, mycodermatitis, narcolepsy, photophobia).

21. Which of the following specialties deals particularly with problems of the elderly? (cryosurgery, gerontology, oncology, orthodontics)
22. A fever-producing agent is called a (pyoderma, pyogen, pyrogen, pyrophobia).
23. Which of the following terms does *not* contain a word part that indicates large or enlarged? (cardiomegaly, macrocephaly, microorganism, megalocyte)
24. The term *electroencephalograph* has something to do with recording the electrical impulses of the brain. Specifically, the term refers to the (instrument used, outcome, process itself, record produced).

Chapter 4

25. A deficiency of white blood cells is (erythrocytosis, hemolysis, leukopenia, cyanosis).
26. A sticking together of two structures that are normally separated is called an (ascites, abdominal paracentesis, adhesion, anuria).
27. Abdominal exploration that uses a special instrument to view the interior of the abdomen is (laparocolostomy, laparohysteropexy, laparorrhaphy, laparoscopy).
28. Measurement of the dimensions and capacity of the pelvis is (cephalopelvic disproportion, pelvimeter, pelvimetry, umbilical).
29. Surgical puncture of the chest wall for aspiration of fluids is (thoracic, thoracentesis, thoracodynia, thoracoplasty).
30. Congenital hernia of the navel is (omphalitis, omphalorrhexis, omphalorrhagia, omphalocele).
31. A headache is (cephalodynia, hematoma, lacrimation, peritonitis).
32. Sagging of the eyelid is (blepharal, blepharedema, blepharitis, blepharoptosis).
33. Inflammation of the skin of the arms and legs is (acrocyanosis, acrodermatitis, acrohypothermy, acromegaly).
34. Cramping of a finger or toe is (chiropody, chirospasm, dactylitis, dactylospasm).

Chapter 5

35. Lateral curvature of the spine is (hunchback, rickets, scoliosis, spina bifida).
36. Inflammation of the bone, especially of the bone marrow, is (osteitis deformans, osteomalacia, osteoporosis, osteomyelitis).

37. Excision of cartilage is (chondrectomy, chondrocostal, subchondral, vertebrochondral).
38. Articulation is another name for (fascia, joint, ligament, tendon).
39. Sacs of fluid located in areas of friction, especially in the joints, are called (bursae, fasciae, laminae, septa).
40. Inflammation of more than one joint is (arthrocentesis, arthrodynia, polyarthritis, quadriplegia).
41. Displacement of a bone from a joint is called (dislocation, fracture, sprain, strain).
42. Pulling the broken ends of a bone into alignment by manipulation without surgery is called (closed reduction, compound fracture, open reduction, simple fracture).
43. A weakness in the abdominal wall resulting in the protrusion of a hernial sac that contains part of the intestine is called (inguinal hernia, multiple myeloma, myocele, polymyositis).
44. A malignant tumor composed of cartilage is (chondrosarcoma, gout, leukemia, sarcoidosis).

Chapter 6

45. Inflammation of the lining of the heart is (endocarditis, polyarteritis, myocarditis, pericarditis).
46. (Cardiovascular, circulation, hemangioma, interstitial) pertains to the heart and blood vessels.
47. Death of part of the heart muscle is (angina pectoris, congestive heart failure, myocardial infarction, myocardial ischemia).
48. A general term that designates primary myocardial disease is (cardiomyopathy, congenital heart defect, heart block, ischemia).
49. A severe cardiac arrhythmia in which contractions are rapid, uncoordinated, and ineffective is (cardiopulmonary resuscitation, catheterization, coronary heart disease, fibrillation).
50. An excessive quantity of fat in the blood is (hyperkalemia, hyperlipemia, hypernatremia, hypertension).
51. The use of ultrasound for diagnosing heart disease is (cardiac catheterization, computed tomography, echocardiography, electrocardiography).
52. Intercellular or interstitial fluid is the same as (intracellular fluid, plasma, serum, tissue fluid).
53. Ballooning out of the wall of a vessel, usually of an artery, because of a congenital defect or weakness of the vessel wall, is (an aneurysm, an embolus, a hemorrhoid, a thrombus).
54. The sudden blocking of an artery or lymph vessel by foreign material that has been brought by the circulating blood is known as (arteritis, embolism, lymphedema, varicosity).

55. A substance that delays or prevents blood from clotting is (an anticoagulant, a coagulation, a phagocyte, a thrombocyte).

56. Cells that can ingest and destroy particulate substances are called (erythrocytes, phagocytes, sickle cells, thrombocytes).

57. The fluid transported by lymphatic vessels is (lymph, lymphoma, plasma, serum).

58. Any disease of the lymph nodes is a (lymphadenitis, lymphadenopathy, lymphadenoma, lymphangiography).

Chapter 7

59. Labored or difficult breathing is (bradypnea, dyspnea, hyperpnea, tachypnea).

60. Which of the following is a machine for prolonged artificial respiration? (expirator, ventilator, spirometer, thoracometer)

61. (Pneumatic, pneumohemothorax, pnemonectomy, pneumothorax) is removal of lung tissue.

62. The sudden blocking of an artery by foreign material is called (edema, embolism, lobectomy, pleurisy).

63. Rhinitis is inflammation of the (chest, nose, throat, voice box).

64. Pulmonary refers to the (chest, diaphragm, heart, lungs).

65. Pharyngitis is inflammation of the (chest, nose, throat, voice box).

66. Chronic laryngitis is most likely to cause which of the following? (aphasia, aphonia, olfaction, rales)

67. Material raised from inflamed membranes of the respiratory tract is (emphysema, saliva, sputum, wheeze).

68. An agent that is used to prevent or relieve a cough is a(n) (antitussive, bronchodilator, epiglottis, rhinorrhea).

69. A disease process that decreases the ability of the lungs to perform their ventilatory function, and can result from several other chronic disorders of the respiratory organs, is (COPD, hyaline membrane disease, RDS, TB).

70. A term that means pertaining to the windpipe and the bronchi is (bronchiectasis, laryngobronchial, pharyngobronchial, tracheobronchial).

Chapter 8

71. A condition that results when the output of body fluid exceeds fluid intake is (achlorhydria, dehydration, enterostasis, peristalsis).

72. Which of the following is *not* part of the small intestine? (cecum, duodenum, jejunum, ileum)

73. Which of the following is *not* considered to be an accessory organ of the digestive system? (gallbladder, liver, salivary gland, spleen)

74. Another name for the gum is (gingiva, peristalsis, pylorus, stoma).

75. Washing out of the stomach is called (gastralgia, gastric lavage, gastrodynia, stomal irrigation).

76. The presence of stones in the gallbladder or common duct is (cholangiography, cholecystitis, cholecystography, cholelithiasis).

77. Which of the following is *not* generally characteristic of untreated diabetes mellitus? (glycosuria, hyperglycemia, jaundice, polyuria)

78. Large internal organs of the body are called (anastoma, melena, peritoneum, viscera).

79. Removal of liver tissue by puncturing the skin overlying the liver with a needle is called (open, resection, percutaneous, wedge) liver biopsy.

80. A procedure performed to decrease the amount of gastric juices by severing the nerves that control their release is a (cholecystectomy, colon resection, gastrectomy, vagotomy).

81. An inability to swallow or difficulty in swallowing is (diverticulitis, dyspepsia, dysphagia, lithiasis).

82. Inflammation of a small sac or pouch in the intestinal tract, causing stagnation of feces and pain, is (colitis, diverticulitis, duodenitis, hemorrhoids).

83. A GI series refers to the use of contrast agents to evaluate the (gallbladder, gastrointestinal tract, pancreas, salivary glands).

84. Cirrhosis is a chronic disease of the (gallbladder, liver, pancreas, stomach).

85. Gastrocele means herniation of the (gallbladder, large intestine, liver, stomach).

Chapter 9

86. Enlargement of one or both kidneys is (diuresis, nephromegaly, nephropexy, nephroptosis).

87. Renal pertains to (the bladder, the kidney, urine, urination).

88. A condition in which there are degenerative, but not inflammatory, changes in the kidneys is (catheterization, nephritis, nephrosis, percutaneous nephrostomy).

89. Surgical incision of the kidney to remove a stone from the renal pelvis is (lithotripsy, lithotrite, pyelolithotomy, ureterolithectomy).

90. Blood in the urine is (albuminuria, hematuria, ketonuria, proteinuria).

Chapter 10

91. Reproductive organs are called the (genitalia, gonadotropin, uteri, vulva).

92. Which of the following means within the uterus? (cervix uteri, extrauterine, intrauterine, myometrium)

93. Removal of an ovary and its accompanying uterine tube is a(n) (abdominal hysterectomy, vaginal hysterectomy, salpingo-oophorectomy, tubal ligation).

94. Menopause is also called (amenorrhea, climacteric, dysmenorrhea, fistula).

95. Inflammation of the inner lining of the uterus is (cervicitis, endometriosis, endometritis, vaginitis).

96. A surgical procedure that expands the cervical opening so that the uterine wall can be scraped is called (conization of the cervix, dilation and curettage, hysterectomy, laparoscopy).

97. Vaginal is (a noun that means the birth canal, an adjective that refers to the birth canal, a noun that means the womb, an adjective that refers to the womb).

98. An abnormal tubelike passage is a(n) (adhesion, colposcopy, fistula, polyp).

99. Prolapse of the uterus is (endometriosis, endometritis, hysteroptosis, salpingocele).

100. Inflammation of the external female genital structure is (colpitis, urethrovaginitis, vaginitis, vulvitis).

101. Childbirth is (gestation, neonatality, obstetrics, parturition).

102. The abnormal implantation of an embryo outside the uterus is a(n) (ectopic, intrauterine, prenatal, postnatal) pregnancy.

103. A tumor found on a mucous membrane is a(n) (curettage, ovum, Pap, polyp).

104. Surgical rupture of the fetal membranes is (amnion, amniotomy, colporrhaphy, cesarean section).

105. The study of diseases of the female reproductive organs is (gynecology, obstetrics, orchidism, penology).

106. Which of the following abbreviations is a test for early diagnosis of cancer of the uterus? (Pap, PID, TUR, TURP)

107. Excessive flow during menstruation is (dysmenorrhea, menorrhagia, menses, metrorrhagia).

108. Surgical removal of the end of the foreskin of the penis is (castration, circumcision, episiotomy, orchiectomy).

109. A word that means after childbirth is (antepartum, bipara, postpartum, unipara).

110. A hormone that is important in the development and maintenance of male sexual characteristics is (estrogen, chorionic gonadotropin, progesterone, testosterone).

111. Which of the following provides an image of the developing fetus? (amniocentesis, colposcopy, laparoscopy, ultrasonography)

112. Removal of all or a section of the ductus deferens is (orchidoplasty, orchiopexy, vasectomy, vasoplasty).

113. A serous tumor of the testis is called a(n) (hydrocele, metastasis, orchitis, phimosis).

114. Which of the following is a characteristic of early syphilis? (chancre, gonococcus, heavy discharge, immunodeficiency)

115. An STD characterized by blisters on the genital organs is (AIDS, gonorrhea, herpes genitalis, male urethritis).

IV. Writing Medical Terms

Write the word for which each meaning or description is given:

Chapter 2

1. surgical repair of the ear _____

2. inflammation of the appendix _____

3. surgical crushing of a nerve _____

4. surgical removal of the tonsils _____

5. specialist in nervous system diseases _____

6. enzyme that acts on lactose _____

7. hemorrhage from the eye _____

Chapter 3

8. study of fungi _____

9. cancerous tumor _____

10. surgical crushing of a stone _____

11. abnormal preoccupation with fire _____

12. any disease of the eye _____

13. study of cells _____

14. origin or beginning of cancer _____

15. paralysis of all four extremities _____

Chapter 4

16. incision of the chest wall _____

17. measurement of the head _____

18. inflammation of the eyelid _____

19. surgical repair of the hand _____

20. inflammation of the bones of the fingers or toes

_____

21. morbid softening of the nails _____

Chapter 5

22. surgical repair of the skull _____

23. excision of a rib _____

24. visualization of the interior of a joint _____

25. inflammation of a joint _____

26. incision of the cranium _____

27. below the breastbone _____

28. pertaining to a rib and vertebra _____

29. branch of medicine specializing in the skeletal and muscular

systems _____

Chapter 6

30. enlarged heart _____

31. elevated blood pressure _____

32. increased pulse rate _____

33. inflammation of the aorta _____

34. hardening of the arteries _____

35. development or formation of a thrombus _____

36. excision of the spleen _____

37. inflammation of the lymphatic vessels _____

Chapter 7

38. respiratory condition in which there is discomfort in breathing in

any position except sitting erect or standing _____

39. inflammation of the pleura _____

40. pertaining to the air sacs of the lung _____

41. radiography of the bronchi after injection of a radiopaque substance _____

42. inflammation of a sinus, especially of a paranasal sinus _____

43. examination of the interior of the larynx _____

44. plastic surgery of the nose _____

45. chronic dilation of the bronchi _____

Chapter 8

46. loss of appetite for food _____

47. excessive vomiting _____

48. pertaining to the esophagus _____

49. pertaining to the stomach _____

50. stoppage of bile excretion _____

51. enlargement of the liver _____

52. inflammation of the gallbladder _____

53. removal of the vermiform appendix _____

54. inflammation of the gums _____

55. x-ray examination of the gallbladder _____

56. inflammation of the liver _____

57. abnormally low blood sugar level _____

Chapter 9

58. pertaining to the kidney _____

59. inflammation of the renal pelvis _____

60. surgical repair of a ureter _____

61. pertaining to the urethra _____

62. absence of urination _____

63. formation of a new opening into the bladder _____

64. branch of medicine concerned with the urinary tract in both sexes and with the male genital tract _____

65. examination of the urinary bladder _____

66. pertaining to a ureter _____

67. sugar in the urine _____

68. destructive to kidney tissue _____

Chapter 10

69. developing human in utero after 8 weeks _____

70. pertaining to the ovaries _____

71. inflammation of the vagina and cervix _____

72. surgical removal of the uterus _____

73. inflammation of an ovary _____

74. absence of menstrual flow (when normally expected)

_____

75. plastic surgery of the vagina _____

76. surgical opening of the abdomen _____

77. excision of a uterine tube _____

78. newborn infant _____

Physician Specialties

Name	Area of Specialty
Aerospace medicine	Physiologic and pathologic problems encountered by humans in the area beyond the earth's atmosphere
Allergy	Hypersensitivity to allergen(s)
Anatomic pathology	Tissues and organs removed during surgery or autopsy
Anesthesiology	Administration of anesthetic(s)
Cardiology	Heart
Clinical pathology	Clinical laboratory
Dermatology	Skin
Emergency medicine	Trauma and emergency situations
Endocrinology	Endocrine glands and hormones
Epidemiology	Relationship of frequency and distribution of diseases; determination of cause of localized outbreak of disease
Family practice	Primary health care for persons of all ages
Gastroenterology	Stomach and intestines
General surgery	All types of operative procedures for treating disease
Geriatrics	The elderly
Gynecology	Females, especially their genital and urinary systems
Immunology	Immune phenomena
Internal medicine	Internal body structures
Neonatology	Newborn infants
Neurosurgery	Operative procedures on the nervous system
Nuclear medicine	Use of radionuclides for the diagnosis and treatment of disease
Obstetrics	Pregnancy, labor, and delivery
Oncology	Tumors
Ophthalmology	Eye
Orthopedics	Musculoskeletal disorders or diseases
Otolaryngology	Ear, nose, and throat
Otology	Ear
Pediatrics	Children

Table continued on following page

Name	Area of Specialty
Physical medicine	Use of physical agents such as heat, cold, light, electricity, manipulation, and mechanical devices to treat disease
Plastic surgery	Repair or reconstruction of tissues or organs
Preventive medicine	Prevention of mental and physical illness or disease
Proctology	Rectum and anus
Psychiatry	Mental disorders
Radiation oncology	Treatment of cancer by radiation
Radiology	Use of radiant energy for the diagnosis and treatment of disease
Rehabilitative medicine	Restoration of survival ability after injury or disease
Rheumatology	Rheumatic disorders
Sports medicine	Prevention, diagnosis, and treatment of sports injuries
Surgical specialties	Operative methods restricted to certain areas or systems (e.g., cardiovascular, colorectal, head and neck, neurologic, thoracic, urologic, vascular)
Urology	Urinary tract

II

Forming Plurals of Medical Words

Plurals of many medical words are formed using the rules you already know:

1. Some terms only require adding an *s* to the singular noun, as in laceration, abrasion, and analgesic.

2. Many singular nouns that end in *s* or *ch* form their plurals by adding *es*, as in abscess and starch.

3. Singular nouns that end in *y* preceded by a consonant form their plurals by changing the *y* to *i* and adding *es*—biopsy and biopsies, ovary and ovaries.

Use the following table to write plurals of other medical terms. Be aware that there are exceptions to the rules and, when in doubt, it is best to consult a medical dictionary. Some terms also have more than one acceptable plural.

a

If the Singular Ending Is	The Plural Ending Is	Examples
is*	es	diagnosis and diagnoses
um	a	ileum and ilea
us†	i	alveolus and alveoli
a	ae	vertebra and vertebrae
ix‡	ices	varix and varices
ex	ices	cortex and cortices
ax	aces or axes	thorax, thoraxes, or thoraces
ma	mata or mas	sarcoma, sarcomata, or sarcomas
on§	a	spermatozoon and spermatozoa
nx	nges	larynx and larynges

* Some words ending in *is* form their plurals by dropping the *is* and adding *ides*, as in epididymis and epididymides.

† Some singular words ending in *us* form their plurals by dropping the *us* and adding *era* or *ora*, as in the following: viscus and viscera, corpus and corpora.

‡ Certain singular terms ending in *ix* have two acceptable plural forms. The plural of appendix is either appendices or appendixes.

§ Some singular words ending in *on* form their plurals simply by adding *s*, as in chorion and chorions.

III Medical Abbreviations and Symbols

ā before
AB abortion
ABO blood groups
ac before meals (*ante cibum*)
ACh acetylcholine
ACTH adrenocorticotropic hormone
AD admitting diagnosis; right ear (*auris dextra*)
ad lib freely as needed; at pleasure
ADH antidiuretic hormone
ADL activities of daily living
AFB acid-fast bacillus
AHF antihemophilic factor
AI aortic insufficiency
AIDS acquired immune deficiency syndrome
AK above knee
ALL acute lymphoblastic leukemia
ALP alkaline phosphatase (liver function test)
AMA American Medical Association
AMI acute myocardial infarction
AML acute myelocytic leukemia
ANS autonomic nervous system
AP anteroposterior
aq water (*aqua*)
ARDS adult respiratory distress syndrome
ARRT American Registry of Radiologic Technologists
AS left ear (*auris sinistra*)

ASA aspirin
ASD atrial septal defect
ASHD arteriosclerotic heart disease
ATS anxiety tension state
AV atrioventricular
BaE barium enema
BID, bid twice a day (*bis in die*)
BIN, bin twice a night (*bis in nocte*)
BK below knee
BMR basal metabolic rate
BP blood pressure
BPH benign prostatic hypertrophy
BR bathroom or bed rest
BSA body surface area
BUN blood urea nitrogen
BX, bx biopsy
c̄ with
C calorie (large), Celsius, centigrade
C1, C2, etc. cervical vertebrae
Ca calcium
CA cancer, chronologic age
CAD coronary artery disease
CAT computed axial tomography (also called CT)
CBC complete blood count
cc cubic centimeter
CDC Centers for Disease Control

259

CHD coronary heart disease
CICU cardiology intensive care unit
CLL chronic lymphocytic leukemia
CML chronic myelocytic leukemia
CNS central nervous system
COLD chronic obstructive lung disease
COPD chronic obstructive pulmonary disease
CPD cephalopelvic disproportion
CPR cardiopulmonary resuscitation
CRF chronic renal failure
CS central service, central supply; cesarean section
C section cesarean section
CSF cerebrospinal fluid
CSM cerebrospinal meningitis
CT computed tomography (also called CAT)
CUG cystourethrogram
CVA costovertebral angle; cerebrovascular accident
CVOD cerebrovascular obstructive disease
CXR chest x-ray
cysto cystoscopic exam
D & C dilation and curettage
diff differential count (WBCs)
DIP distal interphalangeal
DIPJ distal interphalangeal joint
DIS disseminated intravascular coagulation
DJD degenerative joint disease
DLE discoid lupus erythematosus
DM diabetes mellitus
DOA dead on arrival
DOB date of birth
DT delirium tremens
DTR deep tendon reflex
Dx diagnosis
EAHF eczema, asthma, and hay fever
ECG, EKG electrocardiogram
ECHO enteric cytopathogenic human orphan virus
EEG electroencephalogram
EMG electromyogram
EMI electric and musical induction (brain scanner)
ENT ear, nose, and throat
EOM extraocular movements
ER emergency room
ESR erythrocyte sedimentation rate
F Fahrenheit

FANA fluorescent antinuclear antibody
FHS fetal heart sound
FHT fetal heart tone
FSH follicle-stimulating hormone
Fx fracture
GA gastric analysis
GC gonococcus
GFR glomerular filtration rate
GI gastrointestinal
GP general practice, general practitioner
GU genitourinary
GYN, gyn gynecology
HB, HGB hemoglobin
HCG human chorionic gonadotropin
HCT hematocrit
HgA, HgC, HgE, HgF, HgS hemoglobins A, C, E, F, S
HGH human growth hormone
ht heart; height
H/U history of
Hx history
IC irritable colon
ICU intensive care unit
IgA, IgD, IgG, IgM, IgE immunoglobulins A, D, G, M, E
I & D incision and drainage
IM intramuscular
I & O intake and output
IU international unit
IUD intrauterine device
IV intravenous
IVC intravenous cholangiogram
IVP intravenous pyelogram
jt joint
KJ knee jerk
KUB kidney, ureter, bladder
L1, L2, etc. lumbar vertebrae
LE lupus erythematosus; left eye; lower extremity
LH luteinizing hormone
LLL left lower lobe
LLQ left lower quadrant
LMP last menstrual period
LUL left upper lobe
LUQ left upper quadrant
LPN licensed practical nurse
LS lumbosacral
LVN licensed vocational nurse

MA mental age
MCA middle cerebral artery
MI myocardial infarction
MMPI Minnesota Multiphasic Personality Inventory
MRI (or RI) magnetic resonance imaging
MS multiple sclerosis
MSH melanocyte-stimulating hormone
NGU nongonococcal urethritis
noc, noct night
NPO, npo nothing by mouth (*nulla per os*)
OA occipital artery
OB obstetrics
OB-GYN obstetrics and gynecology
OCG oral cholangiogram
OD once a day; right eye (*oculus dexter*)
omn hor every hour (*omni hora*)
OPS outpatient service
OR operating room
OT occupational therapy
OTC over the counter (drug that can be obtained without a prescription)
p̄ after
PA posteroanterior
Pap Papanicolaou smear, stain, or test
PAT paroxysmal atrial tachycardia
path pathology
pc after meals
PCV packed cell volume
PE physical examination
PEG pneumoencephalography
PICA posterior inferior cerebellar artery
PID pelvic inflammatory disease
PKU phenylketonuria
PMN polymorphonuclear
PMS premenstrual syndrome
PNS peripheral nervous system
po by mouth (*per os*)
PP after meals (postprandial)
PRL prolactin
prn as the occasion arises (*pro re nata*)
pt patient
PT physical therapy; prothrombin time
PTA percutaneous transluminal angioplasty
PTH parathormone
PTT partial prothrombin time
PU peptic ulcer
PVC premature ventricular contraction

PX physical examination
qd every day (*quaque die*)
qid four times a day (*quantum libet*)
R radiology; roentgen
RA rheumatoid arthritis
rad absorbed dose of ionizing radiation
RAIU radioactive iodine uptake
RBC red blood cell
RDS respiratory distress syndrome
REM rapid eye movement
RES reticuloendothelial system
RF rheumatoid factor
Rh rhesus factor in blood
RLL right lower lobe
RLQ right lower quadrant
RN registered nurse
ROM range of motion
RUL right upper lobe
RUQ right upper quadrant
Rx prescription
s̄ without
SA sinoatrial
SC subcutaneous
segs segmented neutrophils
SGOT, SGPT serum glutamic-oxaloacetic transaminase, serum glutamic-pyruvic transaminase (enzyme tests of liver function)
SI sacroiliac
SLE systemic lupus erythematosus
SLR straight leg raising
SNS somatic nervous system
SOB shortness of breath
stat immediately (*statim*)
STD sexually transmitted disease
STH somatotropic hormone
T1, T2, etc. thoracic vertebrae
T_3 triiodothyronine
T_4 thyroxine
T & A tonsillectomy and adenoidectomy
TB tuberculosis
tid three times a day (*ter in die*)
TPN total parenteral nutrition
TSH thyroid-stimulating hormone
TUR transurethral resection
TURP transurethral prostatectomy
U/A urinalysis
UE upper extremity
UGI upper gastrointestinal

URI upper respiratory infection
UTI urinary tract infection
VD venereal disease
VDRL Venereal Disease Research Laboratory
(also test for syphilis)
VO verbal order
WBC white blood cells
WNL within normal limits
XP, XPD xeroderma pigmentosum
= equal or equals
≠ not equal

> greater than
< less than
↑ increase
↓ decrease
+ positive or plus
− negative or minus
± very slight reaction, indefinite
♀ female
♂ male
μ micron
Δ change

IV Pharmacologic Terms, Drugs, and Use

by HARRY E. PEERY*

Pharmacology is the **study of drugs.** A drug is a chemical that has an effect on a living cell or body system.

Drugs include medicines, food additives, environmental pollutants, and poisons. Here we will only be concerned with medicines. Other terms for medicines are **therapeutic drugs** and **therapeutics.**

Therapeutics are used to treat or prevent disorders or conditions, such as infections, upset stomachs, or pregnancy.

Giving a drug to a patient is called drug **administration.** The various ways a drug can be administered are called the **routes of administration.** Drugs can be administered **enterally (orally)** or **parenterally.** Enterally administered drugs are taken by mouth. Parenterally administered drugs are those not given by mouth. Parenteral routes of administration include intradermal, intramuscular, intracardiac, intrathecal, intraperitoneal, intrapleural, intravenous, subcutaneous, conjunctival, and dermal.

Once administered, a drug can remain at the site of administration or it can enter the blood. The movement of the drug from the administration site into the blood is called the **absorption** of the drug. The transportation of the drug to other body tissues is called the **distribution** of the drug. Where and how a drug combines with the

* Modified from Leonard, P.C.: Building a Medical Vocabulary. 2nd ed. Philadelphia, W.B. Saunders, 1988.

tissue is called the **action** of a drug. The results are called the **effect** of the drug. If the effect is confined to the site of administration, the drug has a **local effect.** If it acts on many sites distant from the administration site, the effect is said to be **systemic.** The drug eventually is chemically changed, a process called **biotransformation.**

A measured amount of a drug is called a **dose.** The greater the effect with a single dose, the more **potent** a drug is.

The **generic name** of a drug can be used by any company, whereas the **trade name** or **brand name** is the property of only one company and cannot be used by other companies. The first letter of the trade name is capitalized.

Drugs are grouped into several classes based on their effects. The following list presents most of the classes of drugs and some representative examples. The drugs are listed by generic name, with the trade name in parentheses. The trade name given might be either the only one available or the one more commonly used.

Drug Class	Effects, Uses, and Comments
Analgesic	***Relief of pain***
Narcotic Analgesic	Potential for abuse
Codeine	Mild to moderate pain
Meperidine (Demerol)	Moderate pain
Methadone (Dolophine)	Moderate pain
Morphine	Moderate to severe pain
Propoxyphene (Darvon)	Mild to moderate pain
Non-narcotic analgesic	No abuse potential
Acetaminophen (Tylenol)	Mild to moderate pain
Aspirin (many trade names)	Mild to moderate pain
Phenylbutazone (Butazolidin)	Mild to moderate pain
Anesthetic	***Loss of sensation***
Local anesthetic	Local loss of sensation
Benzocaine (Solarcaine)	Topical anesthetic
Cocaine	Topical anesthetic
Dibucaine (Nupercaine)	Nerve block, spinal anesthetic
Lidocaine (Xylocaine)	Topical anesthetic, nerve block
Procaine (Novocaine)	Nerve block
Tetracaine (Pontocaine)	Spinal anesthetic
General anesthetic	Loss of all body sensation, loss of consciousness
Halothane (Fluothane)	Major surgery
Nitrous oxide	Minor surgery
Thiopental (Pentothal)	Minor surgery, induction anesthetic
Antacid	***Reduction of gastric acidity***
Systemic antacid	Absorbed into the blood
Alka-Seltzer	
Sodium bicarbonate	

Drug Class	Effects, Uses, and Comments
Nonsystemic antacid Gelusil Maalox Mylanta	Remains in the intestinal tract
Anticoagulant	***Prevents clotting of blood***
Indirect-acting	Acts in liver to prevent synthesis of clotting factors
Warfarin (Coumadin) Dicumarol	Can be administered orally or by IV
Direct-acting	Acts in blood to prevent activation of clotting factors
Heparin (Panheprin) Aspirin (many trade names)	
Anticonvulsant	***Prevents seizures***
Diazepam (Valium)	Status epilepticus (continuous tonic-clonic [grand mal] seizure activity)
Phenobarbital (Luminal)	Tonic-clonic, absence (petit mal) seizures
Phenytoin (Dilantin)	Tonic-clonic seizures
Valproic acid (Depakene)	Absence seizures
Antidepressant, Stimulant	***Elevates mood in patients with physiologic depression***
Amitriptyline (Elavil)	Antidepressant
Amphetamine (Benzedrine)	Stimulant
Dextroamphetamine (Dexedrine)	Stimulant
Methylphenidate (Ritalin)	Treatment of hyperkinetic children
Imipramine (Tofranil)	Antidepressant
Antihistamine	***Blocks histamine receptors***
H_1 receptor blocker	Blocks receptors involved in allergic reactions
Chlorpheniramine (Teldrin) Diphenhydramine (Benadryl) Tripelennamine (PBZ)	
H_2 receptor blocker	Blocks the receptors responsible for gastric acid secretion
Cimetidine (Tagamet)	Treatment of ulcers
Antihypertensive	***Reduces hypertension***
Diazoxide (Hyperstat)	Emergency antihypertensive
Hydralazine (Apresoline)	Mild hypertension
Methyldopa (Aldomet)	Mild to moderate hypertension
Propranolol (Inderal)	Mild hypertension
Sodium nitroprusside (Nipride)	Emergency antihypertensive
Thiazide diuretics (many generic and trade names)	Very mild hypertension; used with other antihypertensives in moderate to severe hypertension

Table continued on following page

Drug Class	Effects, Uses, and Comments
Antimicrobial	***Used against microorganisms***
Antibacterial	Bacterial infections
Ampicillin (Amcill)	Gram-positive and some gram-negative
Cephalothin (Keflin)	Mainly gram-positive microorganisms
Chloramphenicol (Chloromycetin)	Gram-positive and gram-negative (broad spectrum)
Chlortetracycline (Aureomycin)	Gram-positive and gram-negative
Erythromycin (E-Mycin)	Mainly gram-positive
Nitrofurantoin (Furadantin)	Urinary gram-negative microorganisms
Isoniazid (Nydrazid)	Antituberculosis
Kanamycin (Kantrex)	Mainly gram-negative, some gram-positive
Nalidixic acid (NegGram)	Urinary gram-negative microorganisms
Penicillin G (K-Cillin)	Mainly gram-positive
Streptomycin	Mainly gram-negative, some gram-positive, tuberculosis organism
Sulfisoxazole (Gantrisin)	Urinary tract — mainly gram-positive
Tetracycline (Tetracyn)	Gram-positive and gram-negative (broad spectrum)
Antifungal	Treatment of fungal infections
Amphotericin B (Fungizone)	Parenteral drug used in severe fungal infections
Griseofulvin (Fulvicin)	Skin fungal infections, such as ringworm and athlete's foot
Nystatin (Mycostatin)	Topical candidiasis infections
Antiviral	Treatment of some viral infections
Amantadine (Symmetrel)	Influenza type A viruses
Antineoplastic	***Treatment of cancer***
Cyclophosphamide (Cytoxan)	
Fluorouracil	
Mechlorethamine (Mustargen)	
Methotrexate (Mexate)	
Vincristine (Oncovin)	
Antiparkinson	***Treatment of Parkinson's disease***
Amantadine (Symmetrel)	Also, antiviral drug
Levodopa (Larodopa)	
Levodopa plus carbidopa (Sinemet)	
Biperiden (Akineton)	
Diphenhydramine (Benadryl)	Also, sedative and antihistamine
Antipsychotic Tranquilizer	***Treatment of Psychoses***
Chlorpromazine (Thorazine)	
Haloperidol (Haldol)	
Lithium (Lithane)	Treatment of manic depression
Thioridazine (Mellaril)	

Drug Class	Effects, Uses, and Comments
Autonomic	*Mimics or blocks autonomic nervous system activity*
Parasympathomimetic	Similar to those of parasympathetic stimulation
Bethanechol (Urecholine)	After intestinal or urinary system surgery, stimulates function of system
Neostigmine (Prostigmin)	Anticholinesterase (blocks the enzyme that breaks down acetylcholine); antidote to pancuronium (Pavulon) neuromuscular blockade; occasionally used to treat myasthenia gravis
Pyridostigmine (Mestinon)	Anticholinesterase; used to treat myasthenia gravis
Edrophonium (Tensilon)	Anticholinesterase; used to diagnose myasthenia gravis
Parasympatholytic	Blocks parasympathetic nerve function
Atropine	Dilates pupils, dries up bronchial secretions during surgery; relaxes bladder in cystitis; antidote for mushroom poisoning and anticholinesterase overdose
Scopolamine	Same as atropine, but has added CNS effect of amnesia; was used for "twilight sleep" delivery; during World War II used as "truth serum," because inhibitions are reduced and information could be easily obtained
Sympathomimetic	Similar to those of sympathetic nervous system stimulation
Epinephrine or adrenaline	Most commonly, treats anaphylactic allergic reactions and stimulates heart activity after cardiac arrest; also used in asthma as a bronchodilator and in various conditions or situations as a vasoconstrictor
Norepinephrine (Levarterenol)	Stimulates cardiac activity and increases blood pressure
Phenylephrine (Neo-Synephrine)	Nasal vasoconstrictor—produces nasal decongestion
Ephedrine (various trade names)	Bronchodilator in asthma; nasal decongestant; mydriatic (pupil dilation); cardiac stimulant

Table continued on following page

Drug Class	Effects, Uses, and Comments
Autonomic (Continued)	***Mimics or blocks autonomic nervous system activity***
Sympatholytic	Blocks sympathetic nerve function
Propranolol (Inderal)	Treatment of hypertension, and cardiac arrhythmias, both of which can be aggravated or caused by excessive sympathetic activity
Cardiac Drug	***Affects the heart***
Digitalis and related drugs	Stimulates heart action without increasing need for oxygen
Digitalis (Digifortis)	
Digoxin (Lanoxin)	
Digitoxin (Crystodigin)	
Antiarrhythmic	Returns heart to normal rhythm
Lidocaine (Xylocaine)	Also, local anesthetic
Procainamide (Pronestyl)	
Propranolol (Inderal)	
Quinidine (Cardioquin)	
Diuretic	***Increases urine production***
Chlorothiazide (Diuril)	
Furosemide (Lasix)	
Spironolactone (Aldactone)	
Hormone Drug	***Mimics or affects endocrine secretions***
Pituitary hormone	
Antidiuretic hormone (Pitressin)	Increases blood pressure
Oxytocin (Pitocin)	Stimulates uterine contractions
Corticotropin (ACTH)	
Growth hormone	Increases body growth
Thyroid hormone	
Calcitonin (Calcimar)	Increases bone formation and uptake of calcium
Levothyroxine (Synthroid)	Synthetic thyroxine (T_4)—increases metabolism
Liothyronine (Cytomel)	Synthetic triiodothyronine (T_3)—acts same as T_4, only faster
Liotrix (Euthroid)	Synthetic T_3 and T_4 in 1:4 ratio; when absorbed, the blood levels will simulate the normal amounts of T_3 and T_4 produced by the thyroid
^{131}I (Iodotope)	Radioactive isotope of iodine—diagnosis and treatment of thyroid disorders
Pancreatic hormone	
Glucagon	Increases blood sugar level
Insulin injection (regular Iletin)	Short-acting form of insulin; treats diabetes by lowering blood sugar level

Drug Class	Effects, Uses, and Comments
NPH insulin (NPH Iletin)	Medium-acting form of insulin
Lente insulin (Lente Iletin)	Medium-acting form of insulin
Adrenal cortex hormone (steroids)	
Dexamethasone (Decadron)	Synthetic anti-inflammatory steroid with minimal sodium retention; prevents cerebral edema during neurosurgery
Fludrocortisone (Florinef)	Synthetic steroid with high sodium retention; treatment of Addison's disease
Cortisol (Cortef)	Anti-inflammatory steroid with moderate sodium retention; used to treat many inflammatory conditions
Prednisone (Deltasone)	Potent synthetic anit-inflammatory steroid; used to treat arthritis and other severe inflammatory states
Ovarian hormone contraceptives	
Diethylstilbestrol (Stilbestrol)	Synthetic estrogen; used to treat some cases of vaginitis and dysmenorrhea; in male, used to treat prostatic carcinoma
Estradiol (Aquadiol)	Main female estrogen
Tamoxifen (Nolvadex)	"Fertility drug"; causes multiple ovulations
Oral contraceptive: Enovid, Norinyl, Ortho-Novum (and many more)	Prevents conception
Testicular hormone	
Testosterone	Aplastic anemia, anemia caused by malignant neoplasms (cancer); cancer of breast in women; male hormone replacement therapy; also, produces euphoria in terminal cancer patients
Synthetic androgens (various trade names)	Develop muscles in both males and females ("body building"); use of such hormones is the only way muscular hypertrophy can occur to such an extent in such a short time; potential for abuse
Labor and Delivery Drug	***Labor and delivery***
Ergonovine (Ergotrate)	Speeds up involution of uterus after delivery
Oxytocin (Pitocin)	Induces or hastens labor

Table continued on following page

Drug Class	Effects, Uses, and Comments
Laxative, Cathartic	***Prevents constipation***
Dioctyl sodium sulfosuccinate (Colace)	Laxative provides mild stimulation, whereas a cathartic produces a more powerful laxative effect, often causing diarrhea; the difference often is determined by the dose given
Milk of magnesia (various trade names)	
Monosodium phosphate (Sal Hepatica)	
Muscle Relaxant	***Causes muscle relaxation, reduces spasms***
Indirect-acting	Causes relaxation by effect on nervous system; also produces sedation
Carisoprodol (Soma)	
Chlordiazepoxide (Librium)	
Diazepam (Valium)	
Methocarbamol (Robaxin)	
Phenobarbital (Luminal)	
Direct-acting	Causes relaxation by effect on muscle
Dantrolene (Dantrium)	Also can treat malignant hyperthermia (a rare side effect of halothane anesthesia)
Neuromuscular Blocker	***In surgery, causes flaccid paralysis so surgeon can cut through muscles without reflex contraction***
Dimethyltubocurarine (Metubine)	
Pancuronium (Pavulon)	Also produces respiratory paralysis in some patients who are on intermittent positive-pressure respirators, as in the treatment of tetanus
Succinylcholine (Anectine)	Most widely used neuromuscular blocking drug in surgery
Respiratory Stimulant	***Stimulates respiration***
Doxapram (Dopram)	Stimulates respiration after surgery in some patients
Sedative, Hypnotic	***Sedative calms a patient; a large dose of a sedative has a hypnotic (sleep-inducing) effect***
Barbiturates	Class of sedatives and hypnotics derived from barbituric acid
Amobarbital (Amytal)	Commonly used longer-acting barbiturate
Pentobarbital (Nembutal)	Most commonly used short-acting barbiturate
Phenobarbital (Luminal)	Most commonly used barbiturate; used also in convulsive disorders

Drug Class	Effects, Uses, and Comments
Secobarbital (Seconal)	Most commonly abused barbiturate
Benzodiazepine	Most prescribed class of sedatives in the United States
Chlordiazepoxide (Librium)	Long-acting sedative
Diazepam (Valium)	Intermediate-acting sedative; also used as muscle relaxant, anticonvulsant, and in cerebral palsy (to relieve spasticity)
Flurazepam (Dalmane)	Short-acting sedative commonly used as a hypnotic in geriatric patients
Other sedatives	
Chloral hydrate (Noctec)	Common sedative and hypnotic
Glutethemide (Doriden)	Sedative that does not produce respiratory depression
Meprobamate (Miltown)	Also used as a muscle relaxant
Methaqualone (Quaalude)	Much abused drug; very rapid acting
Vitamin or Mineral	
Vitamin	Needed in small amounts for normal body function
A	Prevents night blindness
B_1	Prevents beriberi
B_2 (riboflavin)	Prevents anemia; deficiency does not occur alone
B_6 (pyridoxine)	Prevents gastroenteritis, convulsions, neuritis
B_{12} (cyanocobalamin)	Prevents pernicious anemia
Biotin	No known effects of deficiency
C (ascorbic acid)	Prevents scurvy
D	Prevents rickets
E	No known effects of deficiency
Folic acid	Prevents megaloblastic anemia
K	Essential for production of clotting factors
Nicotinic acid (niacin)	Prevents pellagra, which is a syndrome of dermatitis, diarrhea, and dementia
Pantothenic acid	No known effects of deficiency
Mineral	
Calcium	Essential for bone and teeth formation, clotting of blood, and normal nervous system and muscular system activity (including heart)
Iron, available as ferrous gluconate (Fergon), ferrous sulfate (Feosol)	Essential for hemoglobin formation and function of certain enzymes

Table continued on following page

Drug Class	Effects, Uses, and Comments
Vitamin or Mineral (Continued)	
Magnesium	Essential for enzymes to function properly
Manganese	Essential for enzymes to function properly
Phosphorus	Essential for bone and teeth formation and maintaining normal pH of body fluids
Potassium	Essential for normal cardiac and other muscle function, and for nervous system integrity
Sodium	Essential for normal cardiovascular function, maintenance of fluid balance, and nervous system function
Vasodilator	***Dilates blood vessels to increase blood flow through them***
Nitroglycerin (21 trade names)	Treatment of angina pectoris (pain in the chest caused by cardiac ischemia); drug acts by dilating peripheral blood vessels, thus reducing the amount of blood returning to heart and limiting the work the heart must do
Papaverine (Pavabid)	Treatment of cerebral and peripheral atherosclerosis by relaxing smooth muscle of arteries causing vasodilation; this increases blood flow past blood vessels narrowed by disease

V

Glossary of Word Parts

Word Part	Meaning
a-	no, not, without
ab-	away from
abdomin/o	abdomen
-able, -ible	capable of, able to
-ac, -al, -an, -ar, -ary	pertaining to
acr/o	extremities (arms and legs)
ad-	toward
aden/o	gland
adenoid/o	adenoids
aer/o	air
alb/o	white
albumin/o	albumin
-algia	pain
alveol/o	alveolus
amni/o	amnion
amyl/o	starch
an-	no, not, without
an/o	anus
angi/o	vessel
ante-	before
anter/o	anterior, toward the front
anti-	against
aort/o	aorta
append/o, appendic/o	appendix
arteri/o	artery
arteriol/o	arteriole
arthr/o	articulation; joint
-ase	enzyme
atel/o	imperfect

Table continued on following page

Word Part	Meaning
ather/o	yellow, fatty plaque
bi-	two
bil/i	bile
blast/o	embryonic form
blephar/o	eyelid
brady-	slow
bronch/o, bronchi/o	bronchi
bronchiol/o	bronchiole
burs/o	bursa
calc/i	calcium
carcin/o	cancer
cardi/o	heart
carp/o	carpus (wrist)
caud/o	tail, in a posterior direction
cec/o	cecum
-cele	hernia
-centesis	surgical puncture
cephal/o	head, toward the head
cerebr/o	brain; cerebrum
cervic/o	neck, uterine cervix
cheil/o	lips
chir/o	hand
chlor/o	green
chol/e	bile
cholecyst/o	gallbladder
chondr/o	cartilage
-cidal	killing
clavicul/o	clavicle (collarbone)
coccyg/o	coccyx
col/o	colon, large intestine
colp/o	vagina
coni/o	dust
contra-	against
cost/o	rib
crani/o	cranium, skull
crin/o, -crine	secrete
cry/o	cold
crypt/o	hidden
cutane/o	skin
cyan/o	blue
cyst/o	cyst, bladder, sac
cyt/o, -cyte	cell
dacry/o	tear, tearing, crying
dactyl/o	digit (toe, finger, or both)
de-	down, from, removing, reversing
dent/i, dent/o	teeth
derm/a, dermat/o	skin
di-	two
dia-	through
dips/o	thirst

Word Part	Meaning
dist/o	far or distant from the origin or point of attachment
dors/o	directed toward or situated on the back side
duoden/o	duodenum
dys-	bad; difficult
-eal	pertaining to
ech/o	sound
-ectasia, -ectasis	dilatation; stretching
ecto-	out, without, away from
-ectomy	excision
-edema	swelling
electr/o	electricity
-emesis	vomiting
-emia	blood
en-	inside
encephal/o	brain
endo-	inside
enter/o	intestines; small intestine
epi-	above; or upon
erythr/o	red
esophag/o	esophagus
esthesi/o	feeling
eu-	normal; good
ex-, exo-	out, without, away from
extra-	outside
femor/o	femur (thigh bone)
fet/o	fetus
fibr/o	fiber
fibul/o	fibula
gastr/o	stomach
gen/o	beginning; origin
-genic	produced by or in
-genesis	producing, forming
genit/o	genitals
ger/o, geront/o	aged, elderly
gingiv/o	gums
glomerul/o	glomerulus
gloss/o	tongue
glyc/o, glycos/o	sugar
gon/o	genitals, reproduction
gram/o	to record
-gram	a record
-graph	recording instrument
-graphy	process of recording
gynec/o	female
hem/a, hem/o, hemat/o	blood
hemi-	half; partly
hepat/o	liver
hidr/o	perspiration

Table continued on following page

Word Part	Meaning
hist/o	tissue
home/o	sameness
humer/o	humerus
hydr/o	water
hyper-	excessive, more than normal
hypo-	beneath or below normal
hyster/o	uterus
-ia, -iasis	condition
-iac	one who suffers
-ic	pertaining to
ile/o	ileum
ili/o	ilium
immun/o	immune
in-	not
infer/o	lowermost, below
inter-	between
intestin/o	intestines
intra-	within
ischi/o	ischium
-ism	condition, theory
-ist	one who
-itis	inflammation
-ium	membrane
-ive	pertaining to
jejun/o	jejunum
kinesi/o	movement; motion
-kinesia, -kinesis	
lacrim/o	tear, tearing, crying
lact/o	milk
lapar/o	abdominal wall
laryng/o	larynx
later/o	toward the side; farther from the midline of the body or a structure
leps/o, -lepsy	seizure
leuc/o, leuk/o	white
lingu/o	tongue
lip/o	fat; lipid
lith/o	stone; calculus
lob/o	lobe
log/o	knowledge; words
-logist	one who studies; specialist
-logy	study or science of
lumb/o	lower back
lymph/o	lymph, lymphatics
lymphat/o	lymphatics
lys/o	destruction; dissolving
-lysin	that which destroys
-lysis	dissolving, destruction, freeing
-lytic	capable of destroying
macr/o	large

Word Part	Meaning
mal-	bad
malac/o,	soft, softening
-malacia	softening
mamm/o, mast/o	breast
-mania	excessive preoccupation
medi/o	middle or nearer the middle
megal/o	enlargement
-megaly	large, enlarged
melan/o	black
men/o	month
meso-	middle
metacarp/o	metacarpals
metatars/o	metatarsals
metr/i	uterine tissue
metr/o	measure; uterine tissue
-meter	instrument used to measure
-metry	process of measuring
micro-	small
mon/o	one or single
muc/o	mucus
multi-	many
muscul/o	muscle
my/o	muscle
myc/o	fungus
myel/o	bone marrow; spinal cord
narc/o	sleep
nas/o	nose
nat/i	birth
ne/o	new
necr/o	dead, death
nephr/o	kidney
neur/o	nerve
nulli-	none
odont/o	teeth
-oid	resembling
-ole	little
-oma	tumor (occasionally, swelling)
omphal/o	umbilicus (navel)
onc/o	tumor
onych/o	nail
oophor/o	ovary
ophthalm/o	eye
-opia	vision
optic/o, opt/o	vision
or/o	mouth
orchi/o, orchid/o	testes
-orexia	appetite
orth/o	straight
-ose	sugar

Table continued on following page

Word Part	Meaning
-osis	condition
oste/o	bone
ot/o	ear
-ous	pertaining to, characterized by
ovar/o	ovary
ox/o	oxygen
pancreat/o	pancreas
para-	near, beside, abnormal
-para	female who has given birth
par/o	to bear offspring
patell/o	patella (kneecap)
path/o	disease
-pathy	disease
pelv/i	pelvis
pen/o	penis (occasionally punishment)
-penia	deficiency
-pepsia	digestion
per-	through, by
peri-	around
periton/o	peritoneum
-pexy	surgical fixation
phag/o, -phagia, -phagic, -phagy	eating; swallowing
phalang/o	phalanges (bones of fingers or toes)
pharmac/o	drugs; medicine
pharyng/o	pharynx
phas/o, -phasia	speech
phleb/o	vein
-phobia	abnormal fear
phon/o	voice
phot/o	light
phren/o	mind; diaphragm
-plasty	surgical repair
pleg/o, -plegia	paralysis
pleur/o	pleura
poly-	many
post-	after; behind
poster/o	posterior, toward the back
-pnea	breathing
pneum/o, pneumon/o	lung, air
pre-	before
primi-	first
pro-	before
proct/o	anus, rectum
prostat/o	prostate
prote/o, protein/o	protein
proxim/o	nearest the origin or point of attachment
psych/o	mind
-ptosis	sagging; prolapse
pub/o	pubis
pulm/o, pulmon/o	lung

Word Part	Meaning
py/o	pus
pyel/o	renal pelvis
pyr/o	fire
quad-, quadri-	four
rach/i, rachi/o	spine
radi/o	radius; radiant energy
rect/o	rectum
ren/o	kidney
retro-	behind; backward
rhin/o	nose
-rrhage	excessive bleeding
-rrhagia	hemorrhage
-rrhaphy	suture
-rrhea	flow; discharge
-rrhexis	rupture
sacr/o	sacrum
salping/o	uterine tube
scapul/o	scapula (shoulder blade)
schis/o, schiz/o, schist/o, -schisis	split; cleft
scler/o, -sclerosis	hard, hardening
scop/o	to examine; to view
-scope	instrument used for viewing
-scopy	process of visually examining
scrot/o	scrotum
semi-	half; partly
semin/o	semen
ser/o	serum
sial/o	saliva; salivary gland
silic/o	silica
som/a, somat/o	body
son/o	sound
-spasm	twitching; cramp
spermat/o	sperm
spir/o	spiral; to breathe
splen/o	spleen
spondyl/o	vertebra
-stasis	stopping; controlling
stern/o	sternum (breastbone)
stomat/o	mouth
-stomy	formation of an opening
sub-	under
super-, supra-	above; beyond
super/o	uppermost, above
tachy-	fast
tars/o	tarsals (ankle bones)
ten/o, tend/o	tendon
test/o, testicul/o	testicle
tetra-	four
therm/o	heat

Table continued on following page

Word Part	**Meaning**
thorac/o	chest
thromb/o	thrombus, blood clot
tibi/o	tibia
-tic	pertaining to
-tome	instrument used for cutting
-tomy	incision
tonsill/o	tonsil
top/o	place, position
tox/o	poison
trache/o	trachea (windpipe)
trans-	across
tri-	three
-tripsy	surgical crushing
troph/o, -trophic, -trophy	nutrition
uln/o	ulna
ultra-	beyond; excess
uni-	one, single
ur/o	urine; urinary tract
ureter/o	ureter
urethr/o	urethra
-uria	urine; urination
uter/o	uterus
vag/o	vagus nerve
vagin/o	vagina
vas/o	vessel; ductus deferens
ven/o	vein
ventr/o	ventral or belly side
venul/o	venule
vertebr/o	vertebra
vulv/o	vulva
xanth/o	yellow
-y	state, condition

VI

Answers to Exercises

CHAPTER 1

Exercises

I.
1. cyst/o
2. chlor/o
3. an-, supra-
4. -algia, -ase, -ose
5. suffix
6. prefix

II.
1. appendicitis
2. enteral
3. antianxiety
4. antiseptic
5. leukocyte
6. prefix
7. hyperemia
8. endarterectomy
9. endocardial
10. esophagogastrostomy

CHAPTER 2

Exercises

I.
1. H
2. J
3. E
4. I
5. C
6. A
7. G
8. B
9. D
10. F
11. K

II.
1. E
2. F
3. D
4. B
5. G
6. I
7. A
8. C
9. H
10. J

III.
1. -oma
2. -pathy
3. -rrhea
4. spasm
5. -rrhage
6. deficient
7. rupture
8. resembling
9. abnormal fear
10. prolapse

IV.
1. one who
2. specialist
3. enzyme
4. pertaining to
5. sugar
6. condition
7. pertaining to
8. membrane
9. pertaining to
10. capable of, able to

V.
1. tonsillar
2. phobic
3. hemorrhagic
4. microscopic
5. coagulable

Comprehensive Review Exercises

A.
1. hematemesis
2. osteomalacia
3. carcinoma
4. lithiasis
5. colopexy

B.
1. stomy
2. scopy
3. centesis
4. megaly
5. cele
6. rrhexis
7. penia
8. oid

C.
1. discharge
2. cramping
3. excessive preoccupation
4. abnormal fear
5. controlling or stopping
6. one who

D.
1. angioplasty
2. dermatome
3. mastectomy
4. ophthalmalgia
5. angiectasis
6. otic
7. appendicitis

8. tonsillectomy
9. glycolysis
10. coagulable
11. a membrane within the heart
12. dystrophy

E.
1. ophthalmologist
2. otologist
3. neurologist

F.
1. lipase
2. protease, proteinase
3. amylase
4. lactose

G.
1. adenectomy
2. otoplasty
3. neurotripsy
4. ophthalmopathy
5. neurectomy

CHAPTER 3

Exercises

I.
1. red; condition (increase)
2. yellow; condition
3. black; tumor
4. white; skin
5. green; vision
6. white; condition
7. blue; pertaining to

II.
1. electrocardiography, electrocardiograph
2. microscopy
3. hemolysin, hemolytic
4. dermatologist
5. cephalometer
6. carcinogenesis, carcinogenic
7. disease (or pathology)
8. dystrophy

III.
1. movement
2. softening
3. eating or swallowing

4. enlargement
5. hardening
6. eat
7. speech
8. paralysis
9. split
10. movement
11. large
12. split

IV. 1. cancer
2. heart
3. head
4. cell
5. thirst
6. electricity
7. feeling
8. elderly
9. tissue
10. seizure
11. stone
12. sleep
13. dead
14. new
15. tumor
16. light
17. mind
18. pus
19. fire

V. 1. voice
2. place
3. cold
4. straight
5. drugs (or medicine)
6. vision
7. heat
8. air
9. embryonic form
10. hidden
11. fiber
12. fungus

VI. 1. one
2. first
3. part (or half)
4. three
5. two
6. none (or zero)
7. partly (or partially)
8. many

9. many
10. four
11. one
12. below normal
13. excessive
14. large
15. small
16. many

VII. 1. peritonsillar
2. inside
3. away from
4. adductors
5. after, behind
6. middle, behind
7. above
8. before
9. outside
10. under (or below), under
11. between
12. through
13. in (or inside)
14. above
15. above (or upon)

VIII. 1. B
2. E
3. F
4. G
5. D
6. C
7. B
8. C
9. D
10. A
11. C

IX. 1. brady
2. tachy
3. eu
4. in
5. mal
6. ant
7. in
8. dys
9. contra
10. para
11. anti
12. dys
13. para
14. per

15. near
16. hyper

X. 1. an
    2. an
    3. a
    4. an
    5. a

Comprehensive Review Exercises

A. 1. C
    2. A
    3. H
    4. D
    5. B

B. 1. below normal
    2. inside
    3. before
    4. behind
    5. under
    6. not
    7. fast
    8. after
    9. under
    10. upon (or above)
    11. before
    12. above

C. 1. G
    2. A
    3. B
    4. I
    5. E
    6. J
    7. C
    8. D
    9. A
    10. I

D. 1. electrocardiograph
    2. electrocardiogram
    3. electrocardiography
    4. hemolysis
    5. hemolytic
    6. hemolysin

7. cephalometry
8. cephalometer

E. 1. intracellular
    2. euthyroidism
    3. contraindication
    4. dysphonia
    5. oncologist
    6. polydipsia
    7. necrosis
    8. aphasia
    9. tachycardia
    10. narcolepsy
    11. gerontology
    12. pyrogen
    13. microorganism
    14. instrument used

F. 1. cryo
    2. lysin
    3. oma
    4. cyano
    5. kinesio
    6. leuko
    7. necro
    8. itis
    9. dys
    10. phago
    11. scopy
    12. hypo

G. 1. mycology
    2. carcinoma
    3. lithotripsy
    4. pyromania
    5. ophthalmopathy
    6. cytology
    7. carcinogenesis
    8. quadriplegia

CHAPTER 4

Exercises

I. 1. anterior, front
    2. caudal (or caudad), tail
    3. distal, far
    4. dorsal, back
    5. inferior, below

6. lateral, side
7. medial (or median), middle
8. posterior, behind
9. proximal, near
10. superior, above
11. ventral, belly

9. G
10. H
11. I
12. A

II.
1. acr/o
2. eyelid
3. abdomin/o
4. nail
5. periton/o
6. body
7. umbilicus
8. large intestine
9. uterus
10. gastr/o
11. thoracodynia
12. thoracotomy
13. thoracoscopy
14. thoracoplasty

Comprehensive Review Exercises

A.
1. dorsal
2. ventral
3. spinal
4. cranial
5. thoracic
6. abdominopelvic
7. viscera
8. peritoneum

III.
1. eyelid
2. inflammation, blephar
3. paralysis
4. sagging
5. spasm
6. blepharoplasty
7. blepharotomy

B.
1. G
2. E
3. C
4. B
5. F

IV.
1. blue
2. skin
3. extremities
4. heat
5. extremities

C.
1. front
2. back
3. anterior
4. side
5. side
6. middle, side
7. above
8. middle, underside

V.
1. softening
2. tumor
3. nails, fungus
4. onychopathy
5. onychectomy

D.
1. blood
2. white, blood
3. many, urine, condition
4. extemity, pertaining to
5. water
6. blood
7. nail, tumor
8. abdominal wall, incision
9. distant, heart, a record
10. umbilicus, pertaining to

VI.
1. J
2. C
3. D
4. D
5. E
6. F
7. C
8. B

E.
1. leukopenia
2. adhesion
3. laparoscopy
4. pelvimetry
5. thoracentesis

6. omphalocele
7. cephalodynia
8. blepharoptosis
9. acrodermatitis
10. dactylospasm

F.
1. onych
2. dacryo
3. hidr
4. endocrine
5. sialo
6. dacryocyst
7. anemia
8. hemolysis
9. py
10. mucolytic

G.
1. thoracotomy
2. cephalometry
3. blepharitis
4. chiroplasty
5. dactylitis
6. onychomalacia

CHAPTER 5

Exercises

I.
1. J
2. D
3. H
4. I
5. E
6. E
7. F
8. B
9. E
10. G
11. C
12. A

II.
1. femor/o
2. fibul/o
3. humer/o
4. radi/o
5. cost/o
6. tibi/o
7. uln/o
8. vertebr/o, spondyl/o

9. humerus, radius, ulna (3, 4, 7)
10. femur, fibula, tibia (1, 2, 6)

III.
1. cartilage
2. cartilage
3. ribs, cartilage
4. bone, cartilage
5. cartilage
6. chondrectomy

IV.
1. muscle
2. myolysis
3. muscle
4. myopathy
5. muscle
6. muscle
7. muscle
8. muscle
9. muscular
10. pain

V.
1. C
2. D
3. F
4. E
5. B
6. A

VI.
1. F
2. A
3. E
4. B

Comprehensive Review Exercises

A.
1. carpus, carp/o
2. clavicle, clavicul/o
3. cranium, crani/o
4. femur, femor/o
5. patella, patell/o
6. scapula, scapul/o
7. sternum, stern/o
8. tarsus, tars/o

B.
1. cervical
2. thoracic

3. lumbar
4. sacral
5. coccygeal

C. 1. costa
2. phalangeal
3. carpal
4. cranial
5. hematopoiesis

D. 1. E
2. H
3. J
4. F
5. K
6. G
7. A
8. B
9. D
10. J
11. I
12. L

E. 1. crani
2. costal
3. coccyx
4. spondylo
5. herniated
6. carpo
7. tarso
8. oste
9. myelo
10. arthr

F. 1. scoliosis
2. osteomyelitis
3. chondrectomy
4. joint
5. bursae
6. polyarthritis
7. dislocation
8. closed reduction
9. inguinal hernia
10. chondrosarcoma

G. 1. cranioplasty
2. costectomy
3. arthroscopy
4. arthritis
5. craniotomy

6. substernal
7. costovertebral, vertebro-
costal
8. orthopedics

CHAPTER 6

Exercises

I. 1. B
2. A
3. C

II. 1. F
2. J
3. I
4. B
5. G
6. D
7. C
8. A
9. H
10. E

III. 1. (f)ibrillation
2. lipemia
3. cardio
4. scope
5. pacemaker

IV. 1. C
2. D
3. F
4. E
5. A
6. G
7. B

V. 1. D
2. B
3. C
4. A
5. D

VI. 1. arterio
2. aort
3. cardio
4. vascular

5. phleb
6. arteritis

VII.   1. D
2. G
3. C
4. F

VIII.   1. B
2. D
3. B
4. C
5. B
6. D
7. A

IX.   1. anti
2. oma
3. an
4. cyte
5. penia

X.   1. G
2. H
3. F
4. D
5. C

Comprehensive Review Exercises

A.   1. lungs
2. vessel
3. vessel
4. yellow, fatty plaque
5. vein
6. adenoid (or pharyngeal tonsil)
7. sound
8. blood
9. blood
10. muscle
11. spleen
12. blood
13. blood clot
14. sound

B.   1. B
2. B

3. C
4. A
5. D

C.   1. murmur
2. arteritis
3. brady
4. phleb
5. edema
6. angio

D.   1. megalocardia (or cardiomegaly)
2. hypertension
3. tachycardia
4. aortitis
5. arteriosclerosis
6. thrombosis
7. splenectomy
8. lymphangitis

E.   1. endocarditis
2. cardiovascular
3. myocardial infarction
4. cardiomyopathy
5. fibrillation
6. hyperlipemia
7. echocardiography
8. tissue fluid
9. an aneurysm
10. embolism
11. an anticoagulant
12. phagocytes
13. lymph
14. lymphadenopathy

CHAPTER 7

Exercises

I.   1. E
2. C
3. B
4. F
5. A

II.   1. ortho
2. homeo
3. spiro

4. vital
5. ventilator

III.   1. A
        2. E
        3. B
        4. C
        5. D

IV.   1. voice
        2. bronchi
        3. trachea
        4. larynx
        5. nose
        6. pharynx
        7. lung(s)
        8. air
        9. lung
        10. nose

V.   1. itis
        2. broncho
        3. ectomy
        4. phasia
        5. ole

VI.   1. D
        2. E
        3. F
        4. B
        5. C

VII.   1. B
        2. D
        3. E
        4. A
        5. G

Comprehensive Review Exercises

A.   1. F
        2. A
        3. C
        4. B
        5. D
        6. G

B. 1. vital
        2. diaphragm
        3. pleura
        4. heart, lungs (no particular order)
        5. pneumonitis
        6. pulmonary
        7. epiglottis
        8. asthma
        9. emphysema
        10. endotracheal

C. 1. dyspnea
        2. ventilator
        3. pneumonectomy
        4. embolism
        5. nose
        6. lungs
        7. throat
        8. aphonia
        9. sputum
        10. antitussive
        11. COPD
        12. tracheobronchial

D. 1. orthopnea
        2. pleurisy, pleuritis
        3. alveolar
        4. bronchography
        5. sinusitis
        6. laryngoscopy
        7. rhinoplasty
        8. bronchiectasis (or bronchiectasia)

CHAPTER 8

Exercises

I. 1. E
        2. D
        3. H
        4. C
        5. G
        6. B
        7. I
        8. I
        9. H
        10. F

11. A
12. F

II.   1. pancreat/o
       2. hepat/o
       3. periton/o
       4. cholecyst/o
       5. sial/o
       6. bil/i, chol/e
       7. -pepsia
       8. -orexia

III.   1. gastr
       2. colo
       3. vago
       4. cholecyst
       5. ileostomy
       6. gastrostomy

IV.   1. cholelithiasis
       2. cirrhosis
       3. an ulcer
       4. gastrocele
       5. glossitis
       6. diabetes
       7. hemorrhoids
       8. large intestine

V.   1. esophag
       2. enter
       3. stasis
       4. gastro
       5. appendic
       6. cholecyst
       7. hepat
       8. glycemia

Comprehensive Review Exercises

A.   1. F
       2. I
       3. E
       4. G
       5. B
       6. H
       7. D
       8. J
       9. C
      10. A

B.   1. gloss
       2. odont
       3. entero
       4. procto
       5. cirrh
       6. chol
       7. diabetes
       8. lith
       9. stomy
      10. cheilitis

C.   1. dehydration
       2. cecum
       3. spleen
       4. gingiva
       5. gastric lavage
       6. cholelithiasis
       7. jaundice
       8. viscera
       9. percutaneous
      10. vagotomy
      11. dysphagia
      12. diverticulitis
      13. gastrointestinal tract
      14. liver
      15. stomach

D.   1. anorexia
       2. hyperemesis
       3. esophageal
       4. gastric
       5. cholestasis
       6. hepatomegaly
       7. cholecystitis
       8. appendectomy
       9. gingivitis
      10. cholecystography
      11. hepatitis
      12. hypoglycemia

CHAPTER 9

Exercises

I.   1. hemodialysis
       2. diuretic
       3. diuresis
       4. uremia
       5. nephron
       6. urea

II.
1. B
2. A
3. C
4. D
5. E

III.
1. A
2. B
3. C
4. B
5. D
6. E

IV.
1. nephro
2. urethr
3. megaly
4. ureteral
5. pexy
6. glomerulo
7. pyelitis
8. lith
9. cystitis
10. cystoscopy

V.
1. bladder
2. glomerulus
3. kidney
4. cyst
5. renal pelvis
6. urine
7. stone
8. sound
9. kidney
10. urethra

VI.
1. urinary retention
2. anuria
3. cystoscopy
4. nephrosis
5. pyelogram
6. lithotripsy
7. nephrostomy
8. renal pelvis

VII.
1. B
2. D
3. A
4. C

Comprehensive Review Exercises

A.
1. urinary
2. ureter
3. bladder
4. urethra
5. urea
6. uremia

B.
1. F
2. E
3. B
4. G
5. A
6. I
7. D

C.
1. nephro
2. sonography
3. catheter
4. glomerulo
5. polycystic
6. scope
7. litho
8. pyelo
9. cysto
10. uria

D.
1. renal pelvis
2. urine
3. blood
4. stone, or calculus
5. bladder

E.
1. nephromegaly
2. the kidney
3. nephrosis
4. pyelolithotomy
5. hematuria

F.
1. urology
2. cystoscopy
3. ureteral
4. glycosuria
5. nephrotoxic (or nephro-lytic)

G.
1. renal
2. pyelitis

3. ureteroplasty
4. urethral
5. anuria
6. cystostomy

3. B
4. D

VII.   1. bi
2. fetus
3. topic
4. post
5. neo

CHAPTER 10

Exercises

I.   1. E
2. D
3. A
4. B
5. C

II.   1. hyster
2. colpo
3. rrhaphy
4. oophor
5. salpingo
6. ligation
7. laparo
8. dilation, curettage
9. laparo
10. conization
11. speculum
12. gyneco

III.   1. B
2. A
3. C

IV.   1. colpitis
2. endometriosis
3. colposcopy
4. hysteroptosis
5. endometritis

V.   1. birth
2. three
3. none
4. beyond
5. female who has given
   birth
6. sound

VI.   1. C
2. A

VIII.   1. amniotic
2. Down's syndrome
3. amniotomy
4. amniocentesis
5. placenta

IX.   1. E
2. E
3. E
4. G
5. A

X.   1. semen
2. scrotum
3. penis
4. prostate
5. testicle

XI.   1. testo
2. orchi
3. circum
4. vaso
5. ectomy
6. orchid
7. prostat

XII.   1. orchidism
2. prostatic
3. prostatitis
4. orchitis
5. hyper
6. benign

XIII.   1. B
2. A
3. D
4. C

XIV.   1. sexually
2. immune

3. opportunistic
4. coccus
5. syndrome
6. rrhea
7. (s)yphilis

Comprehensive Review Exercises

A.
1. genitals (or reproduction)
2. female
3. neck (or cervix)
4. uterine tissue
5. month
6. serum
7. urethra
8. killing
9. birth
10. sound
11. immune
12. three
13. penis
14. water

B.
1. H
2. G
3. A
4. B
5. D
6. E
7. F
8. C

C.
1. metrium
2. colpo
3. menses
4. salping
5. oophor
6. colp
7. contra
8. gesta
9. spermato
10. orchid
11. crypt
12. prostatectomy

D.
1. genitalia
2. intrauterine

3. salpingo-oophorectomy
4. climacteric
5. endometritis
6. dilation and curettage
7. an adjective that refers to the birth canal
8. fistula
9. hysteroptosis
10. vulvitis
11. parturition
12. ectopic
13. polyp
14. amniotomy
15. gynecology
16. Pap
17. menorrhagia
18. circumcision
19. postpartum
20. testosterone
21. ultrasonography
22. vasectomy
23. hydrocele
24. chancre
25. herpes genitalis

E.
1. fetus
2. ovarian
3. colpocervicitis (also cervicocolpitis or cervicovaginitis)
4. hysterectomy
5. oophoritis
6. amenorrhea
7. colpoplasty (also vaginoplasty)
8. laparotomy
9. salpingectomy
10. neonate

CHAPTER 11

Exercises

I.
1. no, not, without
2. extremity
3. gland
4. air
5. white
6. pain
7. starch

8. no, not, without
9. vessel
10. before
11. against
12. joint
13. enzyme
14. imperfect
15. yellow, fatty plaque
16. two
17. embryonic form
18. eyelid
19. slow
20. cancer
21. heart
22. wrist
23. tail or in a posterior direction
24. hernia
25. surgical puncture
26. head
27. brain (or cerebrum)
28. neck (or uterine cervix)
29. lip
30. hand
31. green
32. gallbladder
33. cartilage
34. killing
35. clavicle (collarbone)
36. vagina
37. dust
38. against
39. rib
40. secrete
41. cold
42. hidden
43. skin
44. blue
45. cyst, bladder, sac
46. cell
47. tear
48. digit (toe or finger)
49. down, from, removing, reversing
50. teeth
51. skin
52. through
53. thirst
54. far, distant
55. directed toward or situated on back side
56. bad or difficult
57. sound

58. dilatation or stretching
59. out, without, away from
60. vomiting
61. blood
62. inside
63. brain
64. inside
65. intestines or small intestine
66. above or upon
67. red
68. feeling
69. normal or good
70. out, without, away from
71. outside
72. stomach
73. beginning or origin
74. aged or elderly
75. gums
76. tongue
77. sugar
78. genitals or reproduction
79. a record
80. recording instrument
81. process of recording
82. female
83. blood
84. half or partly
85. liver
86. perspiration
87. tissue
88. sameness
89. water
90. excessive or more than normal
91. beneath or below normal
92. uterus
93. condition
94. pertaining to
95. not
96. lowermost or below
97. between
98. within
99. condition or theory
100. one who
101. inflammation
102. membrane
103. movement
104. tear, tearing, crying
105. milk
106. abdominal wall
107. seizure

108. white
109. tongue
110. fat or lipid
111. stone or calculus
112. specialist or one who studies
113. study or science of
114. that which destroys
115. dissolving, destruction, freeing
116. capable of destroying
117. teeth
118. vision
119. testes
120. condition (occasionally disease)
121. pertaining to or characterized by
122. near, beside, or abnormal
123. female who has given birth
124. disease
125. eating or swallowing
126. diaphragm or mind
127. after or behind
128. lung or air
129. before
130. first
131. anus or rectum
132. nearest the origin or point of attachment
133. mind
134. lung
135. spine
136. radiant energy or radius
137. behind or backward
138. split or cleft
139. half or partly
140. body
141. sound
142. spiral or to breathe
143. under
144. above or beyond
145. four
146. thrombus or blood clot
147. beyond or excess
148. one or single
149. vessel or ductus deferens
150. state or condition

II.   1. bil/i, chol/e

2. carp/o
3. coccyg/o
4. col/o
5. crani/o
6. -ectomy
7. -edema
8. femor/o
9. fibr/o
10. laryng/o
11. later/o
12. lymph/o
13. -megaly
14. dys-, mal-
15. -malacia
16. mamm/o, mast/o
17. -mania
18. meso-, medi/o
19. macro-
20. melan/o
21. men/o
22. metr/o
23. -meter
24. -metry
25. micro-
26. primi-
27. multi-, poly-
28. muscul/o, my/o
29. myc/o
30. myel/o
31. narc/o
32. nas/o, rhin/o
33. ne/o
34. necr/o
35. nephr/o, ren/o
36. neur/o
37. nulli-
38. -oid
39. -ole
40. -oma, onc/o
41. omphal/o
42. onych/o
43. oophor/o, ovar/o
44. ophthalm/o
45. or/o, stomat/o
46. -orexia
47. orth/o
48. -ose
49. oste/o
50. ot/o
51. ox/o
52. pancreat/o
53. patell/o
54. path/o

55. -penia
56. -pepsia
57. peri-
58. -pexy
59. pharmac/o
60. phas/o
61. phleb/o, ven/o
62. -phobia
63. phon/o
64. phot/o
65. -plasty
66. -plegia
67. -pnea
68. -ptosis
69. py/o
70. pyel/o
71. pyr/o
72. -rrhage, -rrhagia
73. -rrhaphy
74. -rrhea
75. -rrhexis
76. salping/o
77. -sclerosis
78. -scope
79. -scopy
80. semin/o
81. sial/o
82. -spasm
83. spermat/o
84. hyster/o, uter/o
85. spondyl/o, vertebr/o
86. -stasis
87. stern/o
88. -stomy
89. tachy-
90. therm/o
91. thorac/o
92. -tome
93. -tomy
94. top/o
95. tox/o
96. trache/o
97. trans-
98. tri-
99. -tripsy
100. troph/o
101. ur/o
102. colp/o, vagin/o
103. vag/o
104. vas/o
105. ventr/o
106. xanth/o

III.
1. surgical puncture
2. abnormal softening
3. emesis
4. proteolysis
5. otic
6. coloscopy
7. inflammation
8. biopsy
9. angiorrhaphy
10. herniation
11. intracellular
12. euthyroidism
13. contraindication
14. dysphonia
15. oncologist
16. polydipsia
17. necrosis
18. aphasia
19. tachykinesia
20. narcolepsy
21. gerontology
22. pyrogen
23. microorganism
24. instrument used
25. leukopenia
26. adhesion
27. laparoscopy
28. pelvimetry
29. thoracentesis
30. omphalocele
31. cephalodynia
32. blepharoptosis
33. acrodermatitis
34. dactylospasm
35. scoliosis
36. osteomyelitis
37. chondrectomy
38. joint
39. bursae
40. polyarthritis
41. dislocation
42. closed reduction
43. inguinal hernia
44. chondrosarcoma
45. pericarditis
46. cardiovascular
47. myocardial infarction
48. cardiomyopathy
49. fibrillation
50. hyperlipemia
51. echocardiography
52. tissue fluid

53. an aneurysm
54. embolism
55. an anticoagulant
56. phagocytes
57. lymph
58. lymphadenopathy
59. dyspnea
60. ventilator
61. pneumonectomy
62. embolism
63. nose
64. lungs
65. throat
66. aphonia
67. sputum
68. antitussive
69. COPD
70. tracheobronchial
71. dehydration
72. cecum
73. spleen
74. gingiva
75. gastric lavage
76. cholelithiasis
77. jaundice
78. viscera
79. percutaneous
80. vagotomy
81. dysphagia
82. diverticulitis
83. gastrointestinal tract
84. liver
85. stomach
86. nephromegaly
87. the kidney
88. nephrosis
89. pyelolithotomy
90. hematuria
91. genitalia
92. intrauterine
93. salpingo-oophorectomy
94. climacteric
95. endometritis
96. dilation and curettage
97. an adjective that refers
    to the birth canal
98. fistula
99. hysteroptosis
100. vulvitis
101. parturition
102. ectopic
103. polyp

104. amniotomy
105. gynecology
106. Pap
107. menorrhagia
108. circumcision
109. postpartum
110. testosterone
111. ultrasonography
112. vasectomy
113. hydrocele
114. chancre
115. herpes genitalis

IV.
1. otoplasty
2. appendicitis
3. neurotripsy
4. tonsillectomy
5. neurologist
6. lactase
7. ophthalmorrhagia
8. mycology
9. carcinoma
10. lithotripsy
11. pyromania
12. ophthalmopathy
13. cytology
14. carcinogenesis
15. quadriplegia
16. thoracotomy
17. cephalometry
18. blepharitis
19. chiroplasty
20. dactylitis
21. onychomalacia
22. cranioplasty
23. costectomy
24. arthroscopy
25. arthritis
26. craniotomy
27. substernal
28. costovertebral (also
    vertebrocostal)
29. orthopedics
30. cardiomegaly (also
    megalocardia)
31. hypertension
32. tachycardia
33. aortitis
34. arteriosclerosis
35. thrombosis
36. splenectomy

37. lymphangitis
38. orthopnea
39. pleuritis (also pleurisy)
40. alveolar
41. bronchography
42. sinusitis
43. laryngoscopy
44. rhinoplasty
45. bronchiectasis (also bronchiectasia)
46. anorexia
47. hyperemesis
48. esophageal
49. gastric
50. cholestasis
51. hepatomegaly
52. cholecystitis
53. appendectomy
54. gingivitis
55. cholecystography
56. hepatitis
57. hypoglycemia
58. renal
59. pyelitis
60. ureteroplasty
61. urethral
62. anuria
63. cystostomy
64. urology
65. cystoscopy
66. ureteral
67. glycosuria
68. nephrolytic (also nephrotoxic)
69. fetus
70. ovarian
71. colpocervicitis (also cervicocolpitis, or cervicovaginitis)
72. hysterectomy
73. oophoritis
74. amenorrhea
75. colpoplasty
76. laparotomy
77. salpingectomy
78. neonate

Bibliography

Beekley Hospital Systems: *Beekley Coding Guide.* Farmington, CT, Beekley Corporation, 1985.

Boyles, M. V., Morgan, M. K., and McCaulley, M. H.: *The Health Professions.* Philadelphia, W. B. Saunders, 1982.

Dorland's Illustrated Medical Dictionary. 27th ed. Philadelphia, W. B. Saunders, 1988.

Dunsmore, C. W., and Fleischer, R. M.: *Medical Terminology, Exercises in Etymology.* 2nd ed. Philadelphia, F. A. Davis, 1985.

Eisenberg, M. S., and Copass, M. K.: *Emergency Medical Therapy.* 2nd ed. Philadelphia, W. B. Saunders, 1982.

Frederick, P. M., and Kinn, M. E.: *The Medical Office Assistant: Administrative and Clinical.* 5th ed. Philadelphia, W. B. Saunders, 1981.

Fuller, J. R.: *Surgical Technology: Principles and Practices.* Philadelphia, W. B. Saunders, 1981.

Griffiths, H. J., and Sarno, R. C.: *Contemporary Radiology: An Introduction to Imaging.* Philadelphia, W. B. Saunders, 1979.

La Fleur, M. W., and Starr, W. K.: *Health Unit Coordinating.* 2nd ed. Philadelphia, W. B. Saunders, 1986.

Leonard, P. C.: *Building a Medical Vocabulary.* 2nd ed. Philadelphia, W. B. Saunders, 1988.

Luckmann, J., and Sorensen, K. C.: *Medical-Surgical Nursing: A Psychophysiologic Approach.* 2nd ed. Philadelphia, W. B. Saunders, 1980.

Miller, B. F., and Keane, C. B.: *Encyclopedia and Dictionary of Medicine, Nursing, and Allied Health.* 3rd ed. Philadelphia, W. B. Saunders, 1983.

Price, S. A., and Wilson, L. M.: *Pathophysiology.* 2nd ed. New York, McGraw-Hill, 1982.

Sheridan, E., Patterson, H. R., and Gustafson, E. A.: *Falconer's The Drug, The Nurse, The Patient.* 7th ed. Philadelphia, W. B. Saunders, 1982.

Sloane, S. B.: *The Medical Word Book.* 2nd ed. Philadelphia, W. B. Saunders, 1982.

Thomas, C. L. (ed.): *Taber's Cyclopedic Medical Dictionary.* 14th ed. Philadelphia, F. A. Davis, 1981.

Tortora, G. J., and Anagnostakos, N. P.: *Principles of Anatomy and Physiology.* 3rd ed. New York, Harper & Row, 1981.

Walter, J. B.: *An Introduction to the Principles of Disease.* 2nd ed. Philadelphia, W. B. Saunders, 1982.

Wyngaarden, J. B., and Smith, L. H.: *Cecil Textbook of Medicine.* 16th ed. Philadelphia, W. B. Saunders, 1982.

Index

Note: Page numbers in *italics* refer to figures.

Abbreviations, 259–262
Abdominal cavity, 80–81, *81*
Abdominocentesis, 83
Abdominopelvic cavity, 80
Abductor, 61
Absorption of drugs, 263
Acquired immune deficiency syndrome
   (AIDS), 224
Acrocyanosis, 87
Acrodermatitis, 87
Acrohypothermy, 87
Acromegaly, 87
Adductor, 61
Adenectomy, 20
Adenoidectomy, 144
Adenoids, 15, 144
Adhesion, 82
Aerosols, 55
Aerospace medicine, 255
AIDS (acquired immune deficiency
   syndrome), 224
Albino, 40
Albuminuria, 200
Alimentation, 171
Allergy specialty, 225
Alveolus, *153,* 161
Amenorrhea, 208
Amniocentesis, 13, 22, 218
Amnion, 22, 218
Amniotomy, 218
Amylase, 34, 178
Amylolysis, 34
Analgesics, 264
Anatomic planes, 74, *74*
Anemia, 92–93, 140
Anesthesia, 51
  spinal, 115
Anesthesiology, 50, 255
Anesthetics, 51, 264

Aneurysm, 135
Angiectasia (angiectasis), 29
Angiectomy, 22
Angina pectoris, 128
Angiocardiography, 134
Angiocarditis, 132
Angiogram, 15
Angiography, 134
Angiomas, 133
Angioplasty, 22
Angiorrhaphy, 22
Ankylosis, definition of, 117
  spinal, 115
Anorexia, 170
Anoxia, 151
Answers to exercises, 281–298
Antacids, 65, 264
Anterior aspect, of body, 76
Anterolateral location, of body, 78
Anteromedian location, of body, 76
Anteroposterior x-ray projection, 76, *77*
Anterosuperior location, of body, 78
Anticoagulants, 140, 265
Anticonvulsives, 65, 265
Antidepressants, 265
Antihistamines, 265
Antihypertensives, 265
Antimicrobials, 266
Antineoplastic drugs, 266
Antiparkinson drugs, 266
Antipsychotic tranquilizers, 266
Antitussives, 160
Anuria, 93, 198
Anus, *170*
Aorta, 134
Aortitis, 134
Aortography, 134
Aortoplasty, 135
Aphasia, 158

301

Aphonia, 54, 158
Apnea, 150
Appendectomy, 13, 179
Appendicitis, 24, 179
Appendix, vermiform, 179
Arrhythmia, 128
Arteries, 132, 134
Arterioles, 132, 136
Arteriosclerosis, 134
Arteritis, 134
Arthralgia, 117
Arthritis, 116
Arthrocentesis, 117
Arthrodynia, 117
Arthropathy, 117
Arthroscopy, 117
Arthrotomy, 117
Articulations, 116
Ascites, 83
Asthma, 160, 162
Atelectasis, 162
Atherosclerosis, 134
Auditory (eustachian) tube, 157
Autonomic drugs, 267–268

Basophils, *142*
Benign tumors, 46
Bifocal lens, 58
Bile, 175, 177
Biopsy, 20
    lung, 162
Biotransformation, 264
Bipara, 215
Blepharedema, 87
Blepharitis, 87
Blepharoplasty, 87
Blepharoplegia, 87
Blepharoptosis, 28
Blepharospasm, 87
Blepharotomy, 87
Blood, cells, 140, *142*
    coagulation of, 140
    composition and function of, 139
    platelets, 141, *142*
    pressure, 128
    transfusion of, 139
    vessels, 132
Body cavities, 80–82
    extremities, 87
    fluids, 88–89
    reference planes of, 74
    skeleton, 100–101, *101*
    structure, 82, *83*
Bone marrow, 105, 112
Bradycardia, 64
Bradyphasia, 64
Bradypnea, 150

Bronchi, *153*, 160
Bronchiectasis, 163
Bronchiole, *153*, 161
Bronchitis, 160
Bronchodilators, 160
Bronchography, 163
Bronchopneumonia, 155
Bronchoscopy, 160, 162
Bronchus, 160
Bursae, 116
Bursitis, 116
Bypass, 129

Calcification, 112
Calcipenia, 30
Calculi, 47
Capillaries, 132, 136
Carcinogen, 44
Carcinogenesis, 44
Carcinoma, 24, 30
    lymphatic, 143
Cardiac arrest, 35
Cardiac catheterization, 129
Cardiac drugs, 268
Cardiologist, 29
Cardiology, 255
Cardiomegaly, 29, 128
Cardiomyopathy, 127
Cardiopulmonary, bypass, 129
    resuscitation (CPR), 130
Cardiorrhexis, 26
Cardiovascular system, 126
Carpals, *101*, 110
Carpectomy, 110
Carpus, *101*, 110
Cartilage, 115
Castration, 220
Cathartics, 270
Catheterization, cardiac, 129
    urinary, 198
Caudad location, of body, 79
Cecum, 176
Cephalad location, 86
Cephalalgia (cephalgia, cephalodynia),
    86
Cephalometry, 44, 48
Cephalopelvic disproportion, 85
Cerebral, aneurysm, 135
    palsy, 16
Cerebrospinal fluid, 115
Cerebrotomy, 21
Cerebrovascular accident, 135
Cerebrum, 16
Cervical vertebrae, 107, *108*
Cervix uteri, 207
    conization of, 211
    definition of, 207

Cervix uteri (*Continued*)
  polyps of, 213
Cesarean section, 218
Chancre, 223
Cheilitis, 183
Chiroplasty, 88
Chiropody, 88
Chirospasm, 29
Cholangiography, 180–181
Cholangitis, 180
Cholecystectomy, 182
Cholecystitis, 181
Cholecystography, 181
Cholelithiasis, 181
Cholestasis, 185
Chondrectomy, 116
Chondrosarcoma, 120
Chronic obstructive pulmonary disease
  (COPD), 163
Circulatory system, 125–145, *127*
Circumcision, 220
Cirrhosis, 180, 185
Clavicle, *101, 104*
Climacteric, 208
Coagulation, of blood, 140
Coccygeal vertebrae, 109
Coccyx, *108,* 109
Colitis, 184
Collagen disease, 119
Colon, 84, *170,* 175
Colopexy, 19
Coloscopy, 19
Colostomy, 18–19, 182
Colpitis, 213
Colpocervicitis, 210
Colpoplasty, 211
Colporrhaphy, 211
Colposcopy, 213
Computed tomography, 130
Congenital heart disease, 128
Congestive heart failure, 128
Continence, 65
Contraceptives, 63, 213
Contraindication, 65
COPD (chronic obstructive pulmonary
  disease), 163
Coronary arteries, definition of, 127
  thrombosis in, 137
Coronary heart disease, 128
Costectomy, 105
Cranial cavity, 80, *81*
Craniectomy, 104
Craniocele, 104
Cranioplasty, 104
Craniotomy, 104
Cranium, *101,* 104
Cryosurgery, 54
Cryotherapy, 53

Cryptorchidism, 55, 222
Curettage, 212
Cyanosis, 41
Cystitis, 196
Cystocele, 198
Cystoscopy, 196
Cystostomy, 198
Cytology, 46
Cytoscopy, 46

Dacryocyst, 90
Dacryocystitis, 91
Dacryolith (tear stone), 90
Dacryolithiasis, 90
Dactylitis, 88
Dactylospasm, 88
Decalcification, 112
Defibrillation, 128
Dehydration, 171
Dental specialties, 173–174
Dermatitis, 50
Dermatologist, 16, 50
Dermatology, 44, 255
Dermatome, 21
Dermatoplasty, 21
Dermatosis, 30
Dermis, 62
Diabetes mellitus, 177, 185
Dialysis, 190
Diaphoresis, 91
Diaphragm, 80, 152, *153*
Diathermy, 62
Digestion, 170
Digestive system, 170–186, *170*
Digit (finger or toe), 88
Dilatation and curettage, 211, 215
Dilation (dilatation), 23
Disk, herniated, 106, 114
Dislocation, 119
Distal location, of body, 79
Distribution of drug, in body, 263
Diuresis, 190
Diuretic, 190, 268
Diverticulectomy, 184
Diverticulitis, 184
Diverticulum, 184
Dorsal aspect, of body, 78
Dorsal body cavity, 80, *81*
Dorsolateral location, of body, 78
Dorsoventral location, of body, 78
Dosage of drugs, 264
Down's syndrome, 218
Drug(s). See also specific types, e.g.,
  Anticoagulants.
  administration of, 263
  effects of, 264
Duodenitis, 184

Duodenum, *170,* 175
  ulcers of, 184
Dyslexia, 63
Dysmenorrhea, 208
Dyspepsia, 181
Dysphagia, 65, 183
Dysphasia, 158
Dysphonia, 65, 158
Dyspnea, 150
Dystrophy, 44

Echocardiography, 130
Ectopic pregnancy, 54, 216
Edema, 23
  pulmonary, 156
Electrocardiography, 43, 130
Electroencephalography, 48
Electrolysis, 48
Embolism, 138
Embolus, 138, 156
Emergency medicine, 255
Emesis, 23
Emphysema, 161, 163
Encephalitis, 16
Encephalocele, 28
Encephalotomy, 21
Endocarditis, 126
Endocardium, 126
Endocrine glands, 90–91
Endocrinology, 255
Endometriosis, 213
Endometritis, 210
Endometrium, 207
Endoscopy, 84
Endotracheal intubation, 159
Enterostasis, 184
Enzymes, 33
Eosinophils, *142*
Epidemiology, 255
Epidermis, 62
Epiglottis, 159
Epilepsy, 51
Erythroblast, 55
Erythrocytes, 45, *142*
Esophagitis, 183
Esophagus, *170,* 174
Esthesiology, 50
Estrogen, 208
Eupepsia, 181
Eustachian (auditory) tube, 157
Euthanasia, 63
Euthyroidism, 65
Excretion, 190
Exhalation, 150
Exocrine gland, 90–91
Expiration, 150
Extremity(ies), 87

Fallopian (uterine) tube, 206, *207*
Family practice specialty, 255
Fascia, 117
Femur, *101,* 111
Fetal monitoring, 218
Fetus, 206
Fibrillation, 128
Fibrolysin, 55
Fibrosarcoma, 120
Fibula, 100, *101*
Fistula, 213
Fluids, body, 88–89
  spinal, 115
Fractures, 119
Fructase, 33
Fructose, 33

Gallstone, 177
Gastralgia, 174
Gastrectomy, 182
Gastric lavage, 174
Gastrocele, 28, 183
Gastrodynia, 174
Gastroenteritis, 184
Gastroenterology, 175, 255
Gastroscopy, 184
Gastrostomy, 182
General surgery, 255
Generic drug, 264
Genital herpes, 223–224
Genitalia, definition of, 206
  female, 206–214
  male, 218–222
Geriatrics, 255
Gerontology, 50
Gestation, 215
GI series, 184
Gingiva, 173
Gingivitis, 173, 183
Glomerulonephritis, 195, 198
Glomerulus, 193
Glossitis, 183
Glottis, 159
Glucose, 48
Glycogen, 48
Glycolysis, 34
Glycosuria, 178, 200
Gonad, 206
Gonococcus, 223
Gonorrhea, 29, 223
Gout, 119
Gynecology, 206, 255

Heart
  disease, congenital, 128
  failure, congestive, 128
  murmur, 129

Hemangioma, 133
Hematemesis, 28
Hematology, 92, 139
Hematoma, 92, 140
Hematopoiesis, 100
Hematuria, 93, 200
Hemiplegia, 58
Hemodialysis, 92, 190
Hemoglobin, 92, 140
Hemolysin, 44
Hemolysis, 44, 92
Hemorrhage, 25
Hemorrhoidectomy, 137, 182
Hemorrhoids, 137, 184
Hepatitis, 180
Hepatomegaly, 180
Hernia, cerebral, 28
  definition of, 23
  fascial, 118
  hiatal, 183–184
  inguinal, 119
Herniated disk, 106, 114
Herpes genitalis, 223–224
Hiatal (hiatus) hernia, 183
Hidradenitis, 91
Hidradenoma, 91
Hidrosis, 91
Histologic compatibility, 50
Histology, 50
Homeostasis, 126, 150
Hormones, 268–269
Humerus, 101
Hydrocele, 222
Hydrophobia, 25, 91
Hydrotherapy, 91
Hyperemesis, 28, 171
Hyperglycemia, 57, 129, 177
Hyperlipemia, 58
Hyperparathyroidism, 65
Hyperpnea, 150
Hypertension, 128
Hyperthermia, 55
Hyperthyroidism, 65
Hypertrophy, 222
Hyperuricemia, 119
Hypnotics, 270
Hypocalcemia, 58
Hypodermic injection, 57
Hypoglycemia, 35, 57, 178, 185
Hypotension, 128
Hypothyroidism, 65
Hypoxia, 151
Hysterectomy, 210, 212
Hysteroptosis, 213

Ileostomy, 182
Ileum, 170, 175

Ilium, 100, 101
Immunodeficiency, 224
Immunology, 255
Incontinence, 65, 199
Infarction, 129, 137
Inferior aspects, of body, 79
Inferomedian location, of body, 79
Influenza, 163
Inguinal hernia, 119
Inhalation, 150
Inspiration, 150
Insulin, 177
Intercostal muscles, 105
Internal medicine, 255
Intervertebral disk, 106
Intravenous pyelogram, 195
Intubation, 159
Ischemia, 129
Ischium, 100, 101

Jaundice, 177
Jejunum, 170, 175
Joints, 116

Kidney. See also Renal entries.
  polycystic disease of, 199
Kleptomania, 24
Kyphosis, 115

Labia majora, 206
Labia minora, 206
Lacrimal glands, 89
Lacrimation, 89
Lactase, 33
Lactation, 35
Lactose, 33
Laminectomy, 114
Laparocholecystotomy, 84
Laparocolostomy, 84
Laparocystotomy (laparocystectomy), 84
Laparogastrotomy, 84
Laparohepatotomy, 84
Laparohysterectomy, 84, 212
Laparohysteropexy, 84
Laparorrhaphy, 84
Laparoscopy, 84, 212
Laparosplenotomy, 84
Laparotomy, 83
Laryngalgia, 159
Laryngitis, 158
Laryngopharynx, 158
Laryngoscopy, 162
Larynx, 153, 159
Lateral aspects, of body, 74
Lateral x-ray projection, 77

Lavage, 174
Laxatives, 270
Leukemia, 40, 93, 120, 140
Leukocytes, 40, 140, *142*
Leukocytosis, 140
Leukopenia (leukocytopenia), 93, 140
Ligaments, 117
Ligation, 212
Lipase, 34
Lipid, 34, 48
Lipoma, 48
Lithiasis, 30
Lithogenesis, 47
Litholysis, 47
Lithotripsy, 14, 198
Lithotrite, 47, 198
Lobe, pulmonary, 156
Lobectomy, pulmonary, 156
Local effect of drug, 264
Lumbar vertebrae, 107, *108*
Lumpectomy, 20
Lung. See *Pulmonary* entries.
Lupus erythematosus, 119
Lymph, 93
Lymph nodes, 143–144
Lymphadenitis, 143
Lymphadenoma, 144
Lymphadenopathy, 144
Lymphangiography, 143
Lymphangioma, 133
Lymphangitis, 143
Lymphatic carcinoma, 143
Lymphatics (lymphatic system), 93, 143
Lymphedema, 143
Lymphocytes, *142*
Lymphoma, 143

Macrocephaly, 58
Malabsorption, 65
Malignant tumors, 46
Malnutrition, 170
Mammography, 16
Marrow, bone, 105, 112
Mastectomy, 16, 20
Mastitis, 20
Mastopexy, 13, 19
Medial (median) aspects, of body, 78
Medical words, plurals of, 257–258
Mediolateral location, of body, 78
Megalocyte, 45
Melanoma, 46
Menopause, 208
Menorrhagia, 208
Menses, 208
Menstruation, 208, 211
Mesoderm, 60
Metacarpals, *101*, 110

Metatarsals, *101*, 111
Metrorrhagia, 208
Microorganism, 58
Microscopy, 13, 44
Microtome, 14
Minerals, 271
Monocytes, *142*
Mucous membrane, (mucosa), 35, 94
Mucus, 93–94, 175
Multiple myeloma, 120
Multiple sclerosis, 58
Murmur, heart, 129
Muscle relaxants, 270
Muscle strain, 120
Muscular dystrophy, 118
Muscular system, 100
Myalgia, 118
Myasthenia gravis, 118
Mycodermatitis, 55
Mycology, 53
Myelitis, 113
Myeloencephalitis, 113
Myelofibrosis, 113
Myeloma, multiple, 120
Myocardial infarction, 129, 137
Myocarditis, 126–127
Myocardium, 126
Myocele, 118
Myocellulitis, 118
Myofibrosis, 118
Myolysis, 118
Myopathy, 118

Narcolepsy, 51
Narcotic, 51
Nares, 156
Nasal septum, 157
Necrophobia, 49
Necrosis, 49
Neonate, 216
Neonatology, 255
Neoplasm, 46. See also *Carcinoma*.
Nephritis, 195
Nephrolithiasis, 194
Nephrolithotomy, 198
Nephromalacia, 193
Nephromegaly, 193
Nephron, 192
Nephropexy, 194
Nephroptosis, 194
Nephrosis, 199
Nephrosonography, 193–194
Nephrostomy, 198
Nephrotomography, 194
Neuralgia, 23, 28
Neurectomy, 20
Neurologist, 33

Neurolysis, 20
Neuromuscular-blocking drugs, 270
Neurons, 58
Neuroplasty, 21
Neurosis, 16, 24
Neurosurgeon, 16
Neurosurgery, 255
Neurotripsy, 21
Neutrophils, *142*
Nuclear medicine, 255
Nullipara, 58, 215

Obstetrics, 215–218, 255
Occlusion, 129
Omphalitis, 85
Omphalocele, 85
Omphalorrhagia, 85
Omphalorrhexis, 85
Oncology, 46, 255
Onychectomy, 88
Onychoma, 88
Onychomalacia, 88
Onychomycosis, 88
Onychopathy, 88
Onychophagist, 88
Oophorectomy, 210
Oophoritis, 210
Oophorosalpingitis, 214
Ophthalmalgia, 28
Ophthalmitis, 27, 89
Ophthalmologist, 16, 32
Ophthalmology, 255
Ophthalmopathy, 30
Ophthalmoplasty, 21
Ophthalmorrhagia, 28
Ophthalmorrhexis, 29
Opportunistic infections, 224
Optician, 55
Optometrist, 53
Oral surgeon, 172
Orchidectomy, 220
Orchiditis, 222
Orchidoplasty, 220
Orchiectomy, 220
Orchiopexy, 221
Orchitis, 222
Orthodontics, 173
Orthodontist, 54, 173
Orthopedics, 100, 255
Orthopedist, 100
Orthopnea, 54, 150
Osteitis, definition of, 111
   deformans (Paget's disease), 120
Osteoarthritis, 26, 115
Osteoblast, 53
Osteochondritis, 116
Osteomalacia, 24, 112

Osteomyelitis, 113
Osteoporosis, 112
Otitis, 16
Otolaryngology, 255
Otologist, 32
Otology, 255
Otoplasty, 21
Ova, 206
Ovulation, 208

Pacemaker implant, 129
Paget's disease (osteitis deformans), 120
Pallor, 140
Pancreatitis, 185
Pancreatolithectomy, 181
Pap smear, 207
Para-appendicitis, 65
Paracentesis, 83
Paranasal sinuses, 157
Paranoia, 24
Paraplegia, 114
Parasympatholytic drugs, 267
Parasympathomimetic drugs, 267
Parathyroid glands, 65
Parenteral administration, of drugs, 263
Paroxysmal attacks, 162
Parturition, 215
Patella, *101*, 111
Pathologist, 32
Pathology, anatomic and clinical, 255
Pediatrics, 255
Pedodontics, 173
Pelvic cavity, 80, *81*
Pelvic girdle, 109
Pelvic inflammatory disease, 214
Pelvimetry, 85
Pelvis, definition of, 85
   of kidney (renal), 193, 195
   structure of, 109
Percutaneous biopsies, 162, 183, 198
Periappendicitis, 61
Pericarditis, 126
Pericardium, 126
Periodontics, 174
Periodontium, 174
Peritoneum, 81, 182, 190
Peritonitis, 83, 182
Pertussis, 160
Phagocyte, 140
Phalanges, *101*, 111
Phalangitis, 111
Pharmacology, 263
Pharmacotherapy, 54
Pharyngeal tonsils (adenoids), 144
Pharyngitis, 157
Pharynx, *153*, 157, 174
Phlebectomy, 137

Phlebitis, 30, 136
Phlebostasis, 30
Photophobia, 49
Physical medicine, 256
Placenta, 215
Plasma, 139
Plastic surgery, 13, 256
Platelets, 141, *142*
Pleura, 152, *153*
Pleural cavity, 152
Pleuritis (pleurisy), 152
Pneumectomy, 155
Pneumocentesis, 155
Pneumoconiosis, 163
Pneumohemothorax, 155
Pneumonectomy, 155
Pneumonitis (pneumonia), 155
Pneumothorax, 155
Polyarteritis, 135
Polyarthritis, 117, 135
Polycystic kidney disease, 199
Polydipsia, 52, 58
Polyp, 199
    cervical, 213
Polyuria, 93, 177, 190
Posterior aspects, of body, 76
Posteroanterior x-ray projection, *77*
Posteroexternal location, of body, 76
Posterointernal location, of body, 76
Posterolateral location, of body, 78
Posteromedial location, of body, 76
Posterosuperior location, of body, 79
Prefixes, for number or measurement,
    55–57
    for position or direction, 59–61
    use of, 5, 40
Pregnancy, ectopic, 54, 216
    tests for, 215
Preventive medicine, 256
Primigravida, 58
Proctologist, 176
Proctology, 256
Proctoscopy, 184
Progesterone, 208
Pronunciation, rules of, 8–9
Prostatectomy, 221
Prostatitis, 222
Protease (proteinase), 34
Proteinuria, 200
Proteolysis, 34
Proximal location, of body, 79
Psoriasis, 23
Psychiatry, 256
Psychogenesis, 47
Psychology, 47
Ptosis, 25
Pubis, 109
Pulmonary biopsy, 162

Pulmonary edema, 156
Pulmonary embolus, 156
Pulse rate, 136
Pyelitis, 195
Pyelogram, 195
Pyelography, retrograde, 199
Pyelolithotomy, 198
Pyelostomy, 198
Pyoderma, 50
Pyogenesis, 49
Pyrogen, 49
Pyromania, 29
Pyrophobia, 29
Pyuria, 94, 199

Quadriplegia, 58, 114

Rabies, 25, 91
Rachialgia, 109
Rachiodynia, 109
Rachitis, 112
Radiation oncology, 256
Radiology, 256
Radiopaque qualities, 135
Radius, *101*
Rectovaginal fistula, 213
Rectum, 175
Reduction, of fracture, 119
Rehabilitation medicine, 256
Renal failure, 190
Renal pelvis, 193, 195
Reproduction, 206
Reproductive system, 205–225
Resection, 221
Respiration, definition of, 150
    organs of, *153*
Respiratory distress syndrome, 163
Respiratory failure, 150
Respiratory stimulants, 270
Respiratory system, 149–165
Resuscitation, cardiopulmonary (CPR),
    130
Retention, of urine, 199
Retrograde pyelography, 199
Rheumatism, 116
Rheumatoid arthritis, 116
Rheumatoid spondylitis, 115
Rheumatology, 256
Rhinitis, 157
Rhinoplasty, 162
Rhinorrhea, 157
Ribs, types of, *106*
Rickets, 112

Sacral vertebrae, *108*, 109
Sacrum, 109

Saliva, 90, 178
Salpingectomy, 212
Salpingitis, 210
Salpingocele, 214
Salpingo-oophorectomy, 212
Salpingorrhaphy, 212
Sarcoma, 120
Scapula, *101*, 104
Scleroderma, 119
Scleroses, 58
Scoliosis, 115
Scrotum, 218, *219*
Sedatives, 270
Seminal vesicles, 219, *219*
Septum, nasal, 157
Sexually transmitted (venereal)
    diseases, 223–224
Shock, 129
Sialography, 90, 181
Sialolith, 90
Sialolithiasis, 181
Sigmoid colon, 176
Sigmoidoscopy, 176, 184
Silicosis, 163
Sinoatrial node, 129
Sinus, 157
Sinusitis, 157
Skeletal system, 99–121
Sonogram, 130
Spasm, 26
Speculum, 207
Spermatogenesis, 220
Spermatozoa, 206, 220
Spina bifida, 114
Spinal fluid, 115
Spinal anesthesia, 115
Spinal cavity, 80, *81*
Spinal cord, 115
Spine, ankylosed, 115
    vertebrae of, 107, *108*
Spirochete, 223
Spirometry, 150
Splenectomy, 144
Splenomegaly, 144
Spondylarthritis, 117
Spondylitis, definition of, 107
    rheumatoid, 115
Spondylomalacia, 107
Sports medicine, 256
Sprain, 120
Sputum, 160
Stasis, 26
Stenosis, 129
Sternal puncture, 105
Sternum, *101*, 104
Stoma, 159
Stomatitis, 172, 183
Stones, 47

Strain, muscle, 120
Stroke, 135
Sucrase, 34
Sucrose, 34
Sudoriferous (sweat) gland, 91
Suffixes, for surgical procedures, 12–14
    for symptoms and diagnosis, 23–26
    use of, 5, 12
Superior location, 78
Suprarenal glands, 61
Surgery, types of, 256
Sweat (sudoriferous) gland, 91
Sympatholytic drugs, 268
Sympathomimetic drugs, 267
Syndrome, 224
Synovial joints, 116
Syphilis, 223
Systemic drug effects, 264

Tachycardia, 64
Tachyphasia, 64
Tachypnea, 150
Tarsals, *101*
Tarsoptosis, 111
Tarsus, 111
Telecardiogram, 79
Tendonitis, 117
Tendons, 117
Tendoplasty, 117
Tenomyoplasty, 118
Testosterone, 219
Therapeutics, 263
Thoracentesis (thoracocentesis), 85, 162
Thoracic cavity, 80, *81*
Thoracic vertebrae, 107, *108*
Thoracodynia, 86
Thoracoplasty, 86
Thoracoscopy, 86
Thoracotomy, 86
Thorax, 104
Thrombocytes, 141
Thrombopenia (thrombocytopenia), 141
Thrombophlebitis, 136
Thrombosis, 137
Thrombus, 136
Tibia, *101*, 111
Tibialgia, 111
Tonsillectomy, 22, 144
Tonsillitis, 17, 144
Trachea, 14, *153*, 159
Tracheostomy, 14, 159, 162
Tracheotomy, 14, 159, 162
Transfusion, of blood, 139
Transurethral resection, 221
Tripara, 58, 215
Tubal ligation, 212
Tubercles, 163

Tuberculosis, 163
Tumors, 46

Ulcer, definition of, 184
  duodenal, 184
Ulna, *101*
Ultrasonography (ultrasound), 130,
  215–216
Umbilicus (navel), 85
Unipara, 215
Urea, 190
Uremia, 190, 196–197
Ureter, *191*, 192
Ureteroplasty, 196
Urethra, *191*, 192
Urinalysis, 200
Urinary retention, 199
Urinary system, 189–201
Urinary tract, 191
Urination, 190
Urine, 200
Urology, 191, 256
Uterine (fallopian) tube, 206, *207*

Vaginal hysterectomy, 212
Vaginitis, 213
Vagotomy, 183
Varicose veins, 137
Vasectomy, 221
Vasoconstriction, 133

Vasodilation, 133
Vasodilators, 133, 272
Vasoplasty, 221
Vasorrhaphy, 221
Vasostomy, 221
Veins, 132
  varicose, 137
Venous thrombosis, 137
Ventilator, 151
Ventral aspect, of body, 78
Ventral body cavity, 80, *81*
Venule, 132, 136
Vermiform appendix, 179
Vertebra, *101*, 105, 107, *108*
Vesicle, 219
Vesicovaginal fistula, 213
Viscera, 182
Vital capacity, 150
Vitamins, 271
Voiding cystourethrogram, 199
Vulva, 206
Vulvitis, 214

Wheeze, 162
Word parts, examples of, 5
  list of, 273–280
  use of, 6–7

X-ray(s), 76–77, *77*